Basic Guide to Infection Prevention and Control in Dentistry

Basic Guide Series

The Basic Guide series addresses key topics of everyday importance to dentists, dental nurses and the rest of the dental team. The books are designed to be practical and are written in an accessible style with full colour illustrations throughout.

The books published under this series are listed below:

Basic Guide to Dental Procedures, 2nd Edition
by Carole Hollins

Basic Guide to Medical Emergencies in the Dental Practice, 2nd Edition
by Philip Jevon

Basic Guide to Dental Radiography
by Tim Reynolds

Basic Guide to Oral Health Education and Promotion, 2nd Edition
by Simon Felton, Alison Chapman

Basic Guide to Dental Instruments, 2nd Edition
by Carmen Scheller-Sheridan

Basic Guide to Dental Sedation Nursing
by Nicola Rogers

Basic Guide to Orthodontic Dental Nursing
by Fiona Grist

Basic Guide to Dental Materials
by Carmen Scheller-Sheridan

BASIC GUIDE TO INFECTION PREVENTION AND CONTROL IN DENTISTRY

Second Edition

Dr Caroline L. Pankhurst
King's College London Dental Institute

Professor Wilson A. Coulter
University of Ulster

WILEY Blackwell

Registered Office
John Wiley & Sons Ltd, The Atrium, Southern Gate, Chichester, West Sussex, PO19 8SQ, UK

Editorial Offices
9600 Garsington Road, Oxford, OX4 2DQ, UK
The Atrium, Southern Gate, Chichester, West Sussex, PO19 8SQ, UK
111 River Street, Hoboken, NJ 07030-5774, USA

For details of our global editorial offices, for customer services and for information about how to apply for
permission to reuse the copyright material in this book please see our website at www.wiley.com/wiley-blackwell

Library of Congress Cataloging-in-Publication data applied for

ISBN: 9781119164982 [Paperback]

Cover image: © Science Photo Library - PASIEKA/Gettyimages
Cover design: Wiley

Set in 10/12.5pt Sabon by SPi Global, Pondicherry, India

1 2017

Contents

Foreword   viii

Preface   ix

Acknowledgements   x

About the companion website   xi

1 Essentials of infection control   1
   Why do we need infection control in dentistry?   1
   Relative risk and risk perception   2
   Risk assessment and the management decision-making process   3
   How to perform a risk assessment in a dental practice   4
   Hierarchy of risk management control   6
   Infection control and the law   7
   Legal acts under which dental practice is conducted   8
   Published standards and guidance   12
   Team approach to prevention of infection   13

2 Communicable diseases in the dental surgery   16
   How infections are spread   16
   Reservoirs and sources of infection   18
   Infectious diseases by route of infection in dentistry   19
   Infectious disease by route of transmission in the dental surgery   20
   Emerging and re-emerging pathogens   28

3 Occupational health and immunization   34
   Occupational health hazards   34
   Building a culture of safety   35
   Organizing staff health in a dental practice   37
   Immunization requirements for dentistry   39
   Protecting women of childbearing age   39
   Occupational vaccines to protect against hepatitis and TB   43
   Health checks and the consequences of blood-borne virus infection   46
   Health clearance   47
   Duty of care to patients   50

4 Sharp safe working in the dental surgery   53
   Why sharps prevention is important   53
   When do sharps injuries occur?   55
   Preventable sharps injuries   56
   How to avoid a sharps injury   56
   Managing sharps injuries and splashes   60

Occupational health risk assessment for BBV exposure   62
Management of hepatitis C exposures   62
Postexposure prophylaxis for HIV and hepatitis B   64
Recording of sharps injuries   66
Clinical governance and accident risk assessment   66

5 Hand hygiene   68
Hands as a source of infection   68
Hands as a source of hospital-acquired infection   69
Hand hygiene and teamworking   70
Hand hygiene technique   76
Hand care and prevention of dermatitis   82

6 Personal protection for prevention of cross-infection   85
Why we wear personal protective equipment   85
The role of gloves   86
Choosing a suitable glove for the task   88
Managing an allergy to NRL gloves   88
Managing latex allergies in patients   90
Masks and when to use them   91
Protective eyewear and visors   95
Protection during cardiopulmonary resuscitation   97
Tunics and uniforms   99
Protective barriers – plastic aprons and surgical gowns   102

7 Sterilization and disinfection of dental instruments   105
Decontamination cycle   105
Why has cleaning become so important?   106
Legal requirements and technical standards for decontamination 107
Where should instrument decontamination take place?   110
Design of dedicated decontamination units   110
Purchasing of dental equipment   117
Cleaning of dental instruments   118
Disinfection of dental handpieces   121
Mechanical cleaning with an ultrasonic bath   124
Thermal washer disinfectors   126
Instrument inspection   130
Dental instrument sterilization   130
Suitability of sterilizer for different loads   130
Sterilizer installation and validation   131
Steam purity and maintenance of water reservoir chamber   132
How do you know your sterilizer is working?   133
Loading the sterilizer   138
Storage of wrapped and unwrapped instruments   138
Single-use items   142
Variant CJD and rationale for single-use items   144
Disinfection of heat-sensitive equipment and hard surfaces 144
Disinfection of dental impressions   146

8   Dental surgery design, surface decontamination
    and managing aerosols   148
    Dental surgery design   148
    Survival of microbes on surgery surfaces   153
    General cleaning   154
    Surface decontamination in the dental surgery   156
    Management of aerosols and splatter   162
    Managing large blood or body fluid spillages   164

9   Management of dental unit waterlines   167
    What are biofilms?   167
    Risk to staff and patient health from dental unit waterlines   168
    Methods to reduce the biofilm   173
    Control of legionellae in the dental practice water supply   180

10 Healthcare waste management   182
    Legislation on hazardous waste disposal   182
    Types of waste   184
    What is hazardous waste?   185
    Clinical waste segregation and classification   189
    Amalgam waste and installation of amalgam separators   193
    Mercury in the environment   193
    Disposal and handling of hazardous waste in the surgery   195
    Safe handling of clinical waste prior to disposal   197
    Bulk storage of waste for collection   197
    Transport of hazardous waste   198
    Benefits of waste segregation   198

11 Transport and postage of diagnostic specimens, impressions
    and equipment for servicing and repair   201
    Legal framework   201
    Collecting specimens   202
    Transport of specimens to the laboratory   203
    Transport restrictions   204
    Fixed pathological specimens   205
    Transporting impressions   206
    Equipment to be sent for service or repair   206

    Appendix   208
    Table A.1 Daily infection control clinical pathway   208
    Table A.2 Decontamination methods for specific instruments
        and items of dental equipment   211
    Table A.3 Examples of hand and hard surface disinfectants
        and dental unit waterline biocides   214

Index   217

Foreword

Infection prevention and control is everybody's business. In the current era where we confront exotic infections practically every few months, the dental practitioner, which includes each and every member of the dental team, has to be highly conversant and current with the principles and practice of infection control.

The second edition of *Basic Guide to Prevention and Infection Control* is a fitting and comprehensive guide to this rapidly and relentlessly evolving discipline. Both authors are doyens and acclaimed experts of their practice and they have left no stone unturned to provide the reader with a most readable, comprehensive and contemporaneous guide to the subject.

Being engaged in infection control seminars and discussions worldwide, what never ceases to amaze me is the rapidity with which new legislation on infection control evolves in various jurisdictions. This necessarily means that the practitioner has to be fully conversant with the up-to-the-minute legislation, and how and why such pronouncements are made by the regulatory authorities. This book could be considered *the* most wide-ranging exposition of the legislative architecture of dental infection control as currently practised in the United Kingdom. It will nevertheless serve also as a masterful guide for any reader anywhere interested in infection prevention and control.

Written in a very lucid style and a logical manner, the book covers all conceivable aspects of infection control ranging from risk assessment to managing amalgam waste. Admirably, the authors accomplish their goal essentially in 200 pages of text and figures!

I enjoyed perusing the narrative and the ample illustrations that complement the lucid text. I wish this book the success it truly deserves!

December 2016   **Professor Lakshman Samaranayake**
DSc (*hc*), DDS (Glas), FRCPath, FDSRCS (Edin),
FRACDS, FDSRCPS, FHKCPath, FCDSHK
Past Dean of Dentistry, and Professor Emeritus,
University of Hong Kong, Hong Kong
Immediate Past Head, School of Dentistry, and Honorary Professor of Oral
Microbiomics and Infection, School of Dentistry,
University of Queensland, Brisbane, Australia
Professor of Bioclinical Sciences, Faculty of Dentistry, Kuwait University
Professor, King James IV, Royal College of Surgeons, Edinburgh (2013)
Founding Editor-in-Chief, Journal of Investigative and Clinical Dentistry

Preface

This book was written as a practical guide to infection control and prevention in dentistry. The principles of infection control and prevention are universal, and are applicable to the same standard whatever your role in the dental team. Therefore. this book was written to be of value for those in training and all members of the dental team delivering primary and secondary dental care.

It is easy to dismiss infection prevention and control as just being about instrument sterilization and hand hygiene. In reality, infection control, if it is to be relevant and effective, has to take into account psychological attitudes, social norms and prevailing geopolitical dimensions, which is what makes the topic so interesting and dynamic. The science and evidence base underpinning infection control are also universal but standards for delivery and guidelines do vary between countries.

Since the first edition of this book, devolution within the United Kingdom has resulted in restructuring of healthcare with, in some instances, nation-specific legislation and guidance. Reference to these variations can be found by following the hyperlinks cited on the companion website, and in the chapter on legislation. We are delighted to acknowledge that we have a community of readers around the world, so throughout the text and on the companion website we have tried to reflect both national and international approaches to health initiatives in infection control and prevention. Therefore, the reader is guided to the major international sources of advice and guidelines on both infectious diseases and infection control initiatives produced by the World Health Organization, the European Centre for Disease Prevention and Control and the Centers for Disease Control and Prevention in the USA.

Acknowledgements

We would like to thank Dr John Philpott-Howard and Mrs Janet Davies for their most helpful comments and insights during the preparation of this book.

About the companion website

This book is accompanied by a companion website:

www.wiley.com/go/pankhurst/infection-prevention

The website includes:

- Interactive multiple choice questions (MCQs)
- Further reading and useful websites
- Videos

Chapter 1

Essentials of infection control

WHY DO WE NEED INFECTION CONTROL IN DENTISTRY?

Dentists and other members of the dental team are exposed to a wide variety of potentially infectious micro-organisms in their clinical working environment. The transmission of infectious agents from person to person or from inanimate objects within the clinical environment which results in infection is known as *cross-infection*.

The protocols and procedures involved in the prevention and control of infection in dentistry are directed to reduce the possibility or *risk* of cross-infection occurring in the dental clinic, thereby producing a safe environment for both patients and staff. In the UK, all employers have a legal obligation under the Health and Safety at Work Act 1974 to ensure that all their employees are appropriately trained and proficient in the procedures necessary for working safely. They are also required by the *Control of Substances Hazardous to Health* (COSHH) *Regulations 2002* to review every procedure carried out by their employees which involves contact with a substance hazardous to health, including pathogenic micro-organisms. Employers and their employees are also responsible in law to ensure that any person on the premises, including patients, contractors and visitors, is not placed at any *avoidable risk*, as far as is reasonably practicable.

Thus, management of the risks associated with cross-infection is important in dentistry. We do not deal in absolutes, but our infection control measures are directed towards reducing, to an acceptable level, the probability or possibility that an infection could be transmitted. This is usually measured against the background infection rate expected in the local population, i.e. the patient,

Basic Guide to Infection Prevention and Control in Dentistry, Second Edition.
Caroline L. Pankhurst.
© 2017 John Wiley & Sons Ltd. Published 2017 by John Wiley & Sons Ltd.
Companion website: www.wiley.com/go/pankhurst/infection-prevention

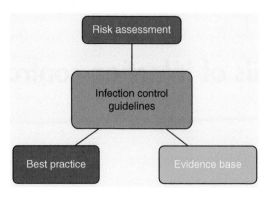

Figure 1.1 Factors influencing the development of infection control guidance in dentistry.

student or member of the dental team is placed at no increased risk of infection when entering the dental environment. Infection control guidance used in dentistry has developed from an assessment of the evidence base, consideration of the best clinical practice and risk assessment (Figure 1.1).

How we manage the prevention of cross-infection and control the risk of spread of infection in the dental clinic is the subject of this book.

RELATIVE RISK AND RISK PERCEPTION

Risk has many definitions, and the dental profession and general public's perception of risk can be widely divergent. This difference in interpretation can impact on how safe the general public perceives treatment in a dental clinic to be, especially following sensational media reports of so-called 'dirty dentists' who are accused of failing to sterilize instruments between patients or wash their hands! For example, risks under personal control, such as driving a car, are often perceived as more acceptable than the risks of travelling by airplane or train, where control is delegated to others. Thus, the public often mistakenly perceives travelling by car to be safer than by air, even though the accident statistics do not support this perception. Unseen risks such as those associated with infection, particularly if they are associated with frightening consequences such as AIDS or MRSA, are predictably most alarming to the profession and the public. Risks can be clinical, environmental, financial, economic or political, as well as those affecting public perception and reputation of the dentist or the team.

What makes risks significant? There are a number of criteria which make risks significant and worthy of concern.

- Potential for actual injury to patients or staff
- Significant occupational health and safety hazard

(Side margin text:) ESSENTIALS OF INFECTION CONTROL

- The possibility of erosion of reputation or public confidence
- Potential for litigation
- Minor incidents which occur in clusters and may represent trends

Understanding what is implied by the term *hazard* is important when we consider the control of infection. This may be defined as a situation, or substance, including micro-organisms, with the potential to cause harm. Risk assessment must take into account not only the likelihood or probability that a particular hazard may affect the patient or dental staff, but also the severity of the consequences.

RISK ASSESSMENT AND THE MANAGEMENT DECISION-MAKING PROCESS

It is the role of managers of dental practices to manage risk. The Management of Health and Safety at Work Regulations 1999 require employers to carry out a risk assessment as an essential part of a risk management strategy. Infection control is an application of risk management to the dental clinical setting.

> Risk management involves identification, assessment and analysis of risks and the implementation of risk control procedures designed to eliminate or reduce the risk.

Risk control in dentistry is dependent on a single-tier approach, in which all patients are treated without discrimination as though they were potentially infectious. The practical interpretation of this concept, known as Standard Infection Control Precautions (SICPs), treats all body fluids, with the exception of sweat, as a source of infection. SICPs are a series of measures and procedures designed to prevent exposure of staff or patients to infected body fluids and secretions. Specifically, dental healthcare workers (HCWs) employ personal barriers and safe behaviours to prevent the two-way exchange of blood, saliva and respiratory secretions between patient and operator (Box 1.1).

Decisions made within an organization, and within practice, should take into account the potential risks that could directly or indirectly affect a patient's care. If risks are properly assessed, the process can help all healthcare professionals and organizations to set their priorities and improve decision making to reach an optimal balance of risk, benefit and cost. If dental teams systematically identify, assess, learn from and manage all risks and incidents, they will be able to reduce potential and actual risks, and identify opportunities to improve healthcare.

Box 1.1 Summary of standard infection control precautions

- Use of hand hygiene
- Use of gloves
- Use of facial protection (surgical masks, visors or goggles)
- Use of disposable aprons/gowns
- Prevention and management of needlestick and sharps injuries and splash incidents
- Use of respiratory hygiene and cough etiquette
- Management of used surgical drapes and uniforms
- Ensure safe waste management
- Safe handling and decontamination of dental instruments and equipment

---

Risk assessment has the following benefits for delivery of dental healthcare.

- Strives for the optimal balance of risk by focusing on the reduction or mitigation of risk while supporting and fostering innovation, so that greatest returns can be achieved with acceptable results, costs and risks.
- Supports better decision making through a solid understanding of all risks and their likely impact.
- Enables dentists to plan for uncertainty, with well-considered contingency plans which cope with the impact of unexpected events and increase staff, patient and public confidence in the care that is delivered.
- Helps the dentist comply with published standards and guidelines.
- Highlights weakness and vulnerability in procedures, practices and policy changes.

HOW TO PERFORM A RISK ASSESSMENT IN A DENTAL PRACTICE

A risk assessment in dental practice involves the following steps.

1. Identify the hazards.
2. Decide who might be harmed, and how.
3. Evaluate the risks arising from the hazards and decide whether existing precautions are adequate or whether more needs to be done.
4. Record your findings, focusing on the controls.
5. Review your assessment periodically and revise it if necessary.

Stage 1: Identify the hazards

- Divide your work into manageable categories.
- Concentrate on significant hazards, which could result in serious harm or affect several people.

- Ask your employees for their views; involve the whole dental team.
- Separate activities into operational stages to ensure that there are no hidden hazards.
- Make use of manufacturers' datasheets to help you spot hazards and put risks in their true perspective.
- Review past accidents and ill health records.

Stage 2: Who might be harmed?

- Identify all members of staff at risk from the significant hazard.
- Do not forget people who only come into contact with the hazard infrequently, e.g. maintenance contractors, visitors, general public and people sharing your workplace.
- Highlight those persons particularly at risk who may be more vulnerable, e.g. trainees and students, pregnant women, immunocompromised patients or staff, people with disabilities, inexperienced or temporary workers and lone workers.

Stage 3: Evaluate the level of risk

- The aim is to eliminate or reduce all risks to a low level.
- For each significant hazard, determine whether the remaining risk, after all precautions have been taken, is high, medium or low.
- Concentrate on the greatest risks first.
- Examine how work is actually carried out and identify failures to follow procedures or practices.
- Need to comply with legal requirements and standards.
- The law says that you must do what is reasonably practical to keep your workplace safe.

A numerical evaluation of risk can be made to help prioritize the need for action and allow comparison of relative risk. *Risk* is equal to *hazard severity* multiplied by *likelihood of occurrence*. Assign a score of 1–5 for each, with a total value of 16–25 equating to *high risk*, 9–15 to *medium risk* and >8 to *low risk* (Figure 1.2).

Stage 4: Record your findings

Record the significant findings of your risk assessment and include significant hazards and important conclusions. Look at how current controls and protocols could be modified to reduce the risk further. Recording can be done simply on a spreadsheet or chart. The most important outcome of any risk assessment is the control measures so focus your efforts on making sure that the control measures the dental practice employs to manage the hazards associated with cross-infection and other aspects of health and safety are sensible and effective.

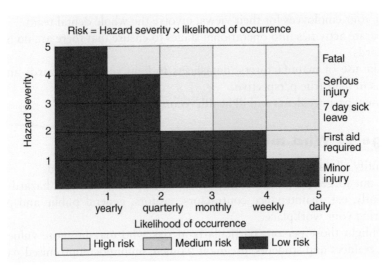

Figure 1.2 Grid showing how hazard severity and likelihood of occurrence are related to risk.

Information to be recorded includes the following points.

- Activities or work areas examined
- Hazards identified
- Persons exposed to the hazards
- Evaluation of risks and their prioritization
- Existing control measures and their effectiveness
- What additional precautions are needed and who is to take action and when

Stage 5: Review your assessment

Risk assessment is a continuing process and must be kept up to date to ensure that it takes into account new activities and hazards, changes in processes, methods of work and new employees.

You must document your findings but there is no need to show how you did your assessment, provided you can show that a proper check was made and you *asked who* might be affected, and that you dealt with all the obvious significant hazards, taking into account the *number of people* who could be involved, that the precautions taken are sensible and reasonable, and that the remaining risk is low.

HIERARCHY OF RISK MANAGEMENT CONTROL

Following a risk assessment, it is necessary to implement a plan to control the observed risk. The plan of action must set out in priority order what *additional controls are necessary*, and aim to reduce risks to an acceptable level and comply with relevant legal requirements. You must also establish a reasonable time scale for completion and decide who is responsible for taking the necessary action.

There is a hierarchy of control options, which can be summarized as:

- elimination (buy in services/goods)
- substitution (use something less hazardous/risky)
- enclosure (enclose to eliminate/control risks)
- guarding/segregation (people/machines)
- safe systems of work (reduce system to an acceptable level)
- written procedures that are known and understood by those affected
- adequate supervision
- identification of training needs and implementation
- information/instruction (signs, handouts, policies)
- personal protective equipment (PPE).

These control measures can be applied as judged appropriate following the findings of the risk assessment, taking into account the legal requirements and standards, affordability and the views of the dental team.

INFECTION CONTROL AND THE LAW

Laws relating to infection control can arise from legal Acts and orders from the individual county or as European Union directives. A distinction must be made between Acts of Parliament, regulations and approved codes of practice and technical advice.

Regulations are laws, approved by the national legislative body. In the UK, the *Health and Safety at Work Act 1974* and in England the *Health and Social Care Act 2008 (Regulated Activities) Regulations 2014* are two primary legislative instruments that embrace all the major regulations, EU directives and technical guidance, for example COSHH, RIDDOR, HTM01-05 (decontamination in primary dental care), HTM07-01 (waste management), etc., that govern the way infection control and cleanliness are achieved in the dental surgery.

The Health and Safety at Work Act and general duties in the management regulations are goal setting and give employers the freedom to decide how to control risks which they identify. However, some risks are so great or the proper control measures so costly that it would not be appropriate to leave the discretion with the employer to decide what to do about regulating them. The Act and Regulations identify these risks and set out specific actions that must be taken. Often, these requirements are absolute – to do something without qualification by deciding whether it is reasonably practicable.

Approved codes of practice (ACOP) offer an interpretation of the Regulations with practical examples of good practice. ACOPs give advice on how to comply with the law by, for example, providing a guide to what is 'reasonably practicable'. For example, if regulations use words like 'suitable and sufficient', an ACOP can illustrate what this requires in particular circumstances. So, if you follow the guidance in the ACOP you will be doing enough to comply with the law. ACOPs have a special *legal status,* which utilizes a reverse burden of proof. 'If employers are prosecuted for a breach of health and safety law, and it is proved that they have not followed the relevant provisions of the ACOP, a court can find them at fault unless they show that they have complied with the law in some other way.'

LEGAL ACTS UNDER WHICH DENTAL PRACTICE IS CONDUCTED

Health and Social Care Act 2008 (Regulated Activities) Regulations 2014

The Health and Social Care Act (HSCA) laid down the framework for provision of new organizational structures and means of commissioning and providing NHS health services in England. The Care Quality Commission (CQC) came into effect on 1 April 2009 and was established by the HSCA to regulate the quality of health and social care. Registration and inspection of dental practices are managed separately in Wales, Scotland and Northern Ireland.

For primary care dental services in England, registration with the CQC as a provider or manager was required from 1 April 2011. It is illegal and therefore a criminal offence for any primary care dental service to carry out any regulated activities unless it is registered with the CQC. Once registered, providers are monitored by the CQC and must comply with any conditions of registration. CQC inspections report on whether the dental services provided are *safe, effective, caring, responsive* and *well led* in relation to a standard set of key lines of enquiry (KLOE), which include 'cleanliness and infection control'. The CQC benchmark for assessing cleanliness and infection control is the HSCA-Approved Code of Practice 2015 which comprises 10 criteria for delivering infection control and prevention across healthcare, including dentistry.

Antimicrobial stewardship in dentistry

Criterion 3 of the HSCA-ACOP relates to antimicrobial stewardship and antimicrobial prescribing. Inclusion of this criterion alongside infection control measures reflects an expedient response to the dramatic rise in antimicrobial resistance worldwide over the last decade, coupled with stagnation in the

> **Box 1.2 Basic principles for antibiotic stewardship in dental practice**
>
> - Systems should be in place to manage and monitor the use of antimicrobials to ensure inappropriate use is minimized.
> - Patients should be treated promptly with the correct antibiotic, at the correct dose and duration whilst minimising toxicity (e.g. allergic reactions) and minimising conditions for the selection of resistant bacterial strains.
> - These systems should draw on published national and local guidelines, monitoring and audit tools, for example: BNF (DPF), NICE, Faculty of General Dental Practice UK guidance on antimicrobial prescribing for general dental practitioners (Open Standards).
> - Providers should ensure that all dental prescribers receive induction and training in antibiotic use and stewardship.
>
> Source: HSCA-ACOP criterion 3.

development of new classes of antibiotics to manage micro-organisms resistant to first-line treatments. In the UK, nearly 70% of dental prescribing of drugs is for antibiotics and research has shown that approximately 50% of dentists overuse antibiotics or are guilty of poor prescribing practices. Box 1.2 outlines the basic principles for setting up antimicrobial stewardship in dental practice.

Health and Safety at Work Act 1974

In the UK, the Health and Safety at Work Act (HSWA) requires a safe working environment and sets the precedent from which all other health and safety regulations follow. Employers have a duty under the law to ensure, 'so far as is reasonably practicable', the health, safety and welfare of their staff and members of the public at their place of work. The HSWA is periodically updated. The *Management of Health and Safety at Work Regulations (MHSWR) 1999* made more explicit what employers are required to do to manage health and safety. MHSWR place the legal responsibility for health and safety primarily with the employer. In particular, this Act required employers to look at the risks in their workplace and take sensible measures to tackle them, i.e. to carry out risk assessments as discussed above. It is the duty of the employer to *consult with staff* on matters which may impact on their health and safety at work, including:

- any change which may substantially affect their health and safety at work, e.g. in procedures, equipment or ways of working
- the employer's arrangements for getting competent people to help him/her satisfy health and safety laws

- the information you have to be given on the likely risks and dangers arising from your work, measures to reduce or get rid of these risks and what you should do if you have to deal with a risk or danger
- the planning of health and safety
- the health and safety consequences of introducing new technology.

The duties of employers under this law include:

- making the workplace safe and without risks to health
- ensuring plant and machinery are safe and that safe systems of work are set and followed
- ensuring articles and substances are moved, stored and used safely
- providing adequate welfare facilities
- giving the information, instruction, training and supervision necessary for the health and safety of staff and the public.

Control of Substances Hazardous to Health Regulations 2002

The law requires employers to control exposure to hazardous substances to prevent ill health. They have to protect both employees and others who may be exposed by complying with the COSHH regulations. COSHH is a useful tool of good management which sets basic measures, with a simple step-by-step approach, that employers, and sometimes employees, must take which will help to assess risks, implement any measures needed to control exposure and establish good working practices.

> Note that hazardous substances include not only chemicals such as mercury, solvents and the materials used in dentistry, but also biological agents such as bacteria and other micro-organisms.

The Regulations require COSHH risk assessment to be made on all the materials used in dental practice.

Under the Regulations, where it is not reasonably practicable to prevent exposure to a substance hazardous to health via elimination or substitution, then the hazard must be adequately controlled by 'applying protection measures appropriate to the activity and consistent with the risk assessment'. Where members of the dental team or students are treating individuals known or suspected to be infected with a micro-organism spread by the air-borne route, then protective measures would include adequate ventilation systems and the provision of suitable personal protective equipment (PPE). The legislation requires employers to provide PPE that affords adequate protection against the risks associated with the task being undertaken. Conversely, COSHH requires that employees actually wear PPE provided by the employer, who should take all reasonable steps to make sure that PPE and any other appropriate control measures are instituted in the practice or dental hospital. The Regulations require risk assessment to be made on all the materials used in dental practice.

Reporting of Injuries, Diseases and Dangerous Occurrences (RIDDOR) 2013

Reporting accidents at work and occupational ill health is a legal requirement. RIDDOR puts duties on employers, the self-employed and people in control of work premises (the Responsible Person) to report to the Health and Safety Executive (HSE) certain serious workplace accidents, occupational diseases and specified dangerous occurrences (near misses). Incidents that happen in Northern Ireland should be reported to HSE NI. This information enables the HSE and local authorities to identify where and how risks arise and to investigate serious accidents. You must report:

- all deaths in the workplace
- specified injuries and over-seven-day incapacitation of a worker which results in the employee or self-employed person being away from work or unable to perform their normal work duties for more than seven consecutive days plus the day of the accident (includes weekends and rest days)
- diagnoses of certain occupational diseases, where these are likely to have been caused or made worse by their work including, for example, Legionnaires' disease, hepatitis B
- non-fatal accidents to non-workers (e.g. members of the public), if they result in an injury and the person is taken directly from the scene of the accident to hospital for treatment to that injury.

The report must be made within 15 days of the accident. Over-three-day incapacitations (but less than seven-day) from accidents in the workplace must be recorded in an accident book but do not need to be reported to the HSE. Thus, the dental surgery must be an environment where we positively encourage accident reporting and near misses by all the dental team.

Pressure Systems Safety Regulations 2000

If pressure equipment fails in use, it can seriously injure or kill people nearby and cause serious damage to property. Because autoclaves are pressurized vessels and are potentially explosive, they come under legal requirements to be tested annually to ensure safety and also for insurance purposes. The Pressure Systems Safety Regulations came into force in 2000 and cover the installation and use of steam sterilizers.

Following installation of the sterilizer and before it is used, the dental practice must obtain a written scheme of examination for each sterilizer from the manufacturer, supplier or insurer that has been prepared by a Competent Person (Pressure Vessels). A certificate is issued as proof of each inspection, and is retained in the sterilizer logbook. Users and owners of pressure systems are required to demonstrate that they know the safe operating limits, principally pressures and temperatures, of their pressure systems and that the systems are safe under those conditions.

As a legal requirement, each sterilizer must have:

- a written scheme of examination
- a periodic examination of the pressure system and retention of the certificate
- third party liability insurance that specifically covers risks associated with the operation of pressure vessels, e.g. sterilizers and compressors. Such risks may not be covered by the practice's building insurance
- a record of all repairs and maintenance of the pressure system.

PUBLISHED STANDARDS AND GUIDANCE

Standards and guidance relating to infection control and prevention are set and can be obtained from a number of government agencies and other public sources. The key agencies and organizations for the UK, and where applicable the country-specific equivalent government organizations and guidance for Northern Ireland, Scotland and Wales, can be found on the companion website (www.wiley.com/go/pankhurst/infection-prevention).

Policy

The arms of government, outlined above, dictate policy which is published in the form of strategic documents which they seek to implement. These policies are often the work of special advisory bodies such as the Advisory Committee on Dangerous Pathogens (ACDP) whose remit is to advise on all aspects of hazards and risks to workers and others from exposure to pathogens and risk assessment advice on transmissible spongiform encephalopathies (TSEs).

When the Department of Health agrees on a strategy, it cascades this down to those local organizations which are tasked with implementation such as local authorities and health boards. Health service circulars and letters from the Chief Dental Officer are used to communicate with people in the dental profession and these can be accessed on the websites for your local area.

Procedures

Guidance and recommendations on infection control procedures undertaken in dental practice are cascaded down to dental professionals via a variety of formats including, for example, health technical memoranda (HTM), health building notes, drug and device alerts, and drug safety updates. These provide the essential information we need if we are to keep up to date with what would be considered good practice. Drug and device alerts are often written in response to adverse incidents where there is a need to communicate changes in practice following from the experience gained when an incident has occurred with equipment or medication.

Health Technical Memoranda

These publications give technical advice and guidance on specific healthcare topics and set out recommendations for good practice. An example of an HTM is *HTM 01-05 Decontamination in Primary Care Dental Practices*, which has had a major impact on dental practice in the UK. This HTM provides in-depth guidance on all aspects of the decontamination cycle, which includes choice, specification, purchase, installation, validation, periodic testing, operation and maintenance of ultrasonic baths, thermal washer disinfectors and sterilizers. The practices and procedures described in HTM 05-01 and the country-specific equivalents are covered in Chapter 7.

Implementation

The implementation of policy and procedures has to be monitored at the local level and this has been incorporated into quality assurance and clinical governance. Clinical governance is a systematic approach to maintaining and improving the quality of patient care within a health system. Governance incorporates existing activities such as clinical audit, education and training, research and development, and risk management. For example, the results of the biannual decontamination audits required under HTM 01-05 act to maintain best practice where it exists, or highlight areas for improvement and generate action plans, steering the move towards best practice in decontamination.

TEAM APPROACH TO PREVENTION OF INFECTION

A team is more than just a group of people working together; it has been defined as:

> A small number of people with complementary skills who are committed to a common purpose, performance goals and approach for which they hold themselves mutually accountable.

ESSENTIALS OF INFECTION CONTROL

Infection control of necessity requires a team approach and each member of the team must have complementary skills and share the common purpose to ensure safe practice. 'For the team to function effectively there must be clear goals shared by the team, good communication between the team members, with clear, fair leadership and an open climate based on respect and absence of a blame culture.' This will encourage staff to feel confident and safe to treat patients with potentially infectious disease and to express their concerns on infection matters and thus contribute to the improvement of service delivery. Generally, teamwork improves job satisfaction, increases the sense of being valued and encourages a collective responsibility for the delivery of service.

Effective leadership is an important constituent of the dental team and leaders (dentists, registered managers or infection control leads) must provide a clear vision of the standard of excellence which the team is seeking to achieve and communicate this to other members of the team. This is best achieved by ensuring that there is adequate induction and ongoing training for all members of the dental team in infection control and that there are regular clinical management meetings within the practice. Meetings are required to allow communication between the team members and for risk assessments to be undertaken as new problems arise. There is evidence that busy dental practices often do not have regular structured team meetings built into their routine, but particularly in the rapidly developing field of infection control, these meetings are essential.

Communication is essential if the members of the dental team are to report accidents and feed back their opinions, reservations and fears regarding infection control policy and conditions of work in the dental practice. Individuals must not be discouraged by the perception of 'failure' if they report accidents or incidents.

It is useful to consider what the causes of human failure are, as human error is one of the most frequent reasons for breaches in infection control practice. Failure is usually caused by either:

- *errors in knowledge* where the HCW did not know what they were supposed to do to, for example, the importance of safe disposal of sharps and the prevention of transmission of infection by aerosol in the clinic, or
- *errors in skills* where the HCW did not have sufficient training to, for example, carry out procedures such as decontaminating an instrument or using a scalpel safely.

There may be a prevailing environment in the dental surgery which, due to poor organization and failure in management, is conducive to personal failure and errors. The reduction of human error is therefore closely related to good practice management and to having an effective team.

Human error can be minimized by improving job design. The employer should ensure that everyone knows his or her duties and has the skills to accomplish the tasks. Prevent boredom and subsequent errors by introducing job rotation and job enrichment. Practices can introduce enhanced training and multiskilling of staff, which gives the HCW new challenges and a sense of ownership and maintains interest and pride in 'a job well done'.

Lastly, encouraging staff participation in decision making and making them feel a valued member of the dental healthcare team will reduce errors, and if errors do occur, they will be quickly corrected and be unlikely to reoccur.

REFERENCES AND WEBSITES

Faculty of General Dental Practice. UK Guidance on Antimicrobial Prescribing for General Dental Practitioners (Open Standards). Available at: www.fgdp.org.uk/publications/antimicrobial-prescribing-standards.ashx (accessed 27 October 2016).

Health and Safety Executive. Risk Assessment – A Brief Guide to Controlling Risks in the Workplace. Available at: www.hse.gov.uk/pubns/indg163.htm (accessed 27 October 2016).

Health and Safety Executive. Control of Substances Hazardous to Health, 6th edn. Approved Code of Practice and Guidance. Available at: www.hse.gov.uk/pubns/books/l5.htm (accessed 27 October 2016).

Health and Safety Executive. Pressure Systems Safety Regulations 2000. Approved Code of Practice and Guidance on Regulations. Available at: www.hse.gov.uk/pubns/books/l122.htm (accessed 27 October 2016).

Chapter 2

Communicable diseases in the dental surgery

HOW INFECTIONS ARE SPREAD

Micro-organizms must attach to or penetrate the surfaces of the body in order to establish themselves and cause infection. This association between microbes and human cells is very specific and has evolved over millennia; thus, many species of bacteria which colonize the mouth and oral tissues are not found anywhere else in the human body or at any other site in the biosphere.

While the body is well protected from microbial invasion by intact skin, the mucosa-lined orifices of the body are sites for potential entry of infection. These sites are protected by secretions such as saliva and tears, and by cellular and antibody immunological defence mechanisms. However, both mucosal surfaces and damaged skin remain a potential weak link in our defences, which is why we wear protective clothing such as masks to protect the respiratory tree, lips and mouth from infection, and goggles to protect the eyes as part of our infection control and prevention protocols.

The vast majority of microbes do not cause infection in humans; indeed, a *resident* or *commensal* flora on the skin, in the gut and mouth is essential for health. These bacteria live in harmony with our body and protect us by competing with other more harmful bacteria and thereby preventing colonization. An example of this is seen in dental plaque. *Streptococcus sanguinis* and the cariogenic mutans streptococci compete for colonization of the infant mouth. The presence of *S. sanguinis* can delay the colonization of the mouth by mutans streptococci with a subsequent reduction in the dental caries rate.

Some microbes which in healthy people are considered commensal and harmless can cause infection if the host's immune system is compromised by,

Basic Guide to Infection Prevention and Control in Dentistry, Second Edition.
Caroline L. Pankhurst.
© 2017 John Wiley & Sons Ltd. Published 2017 by John Wiley & Sons Ltd.
Companion website: www.wiley.com/go/pankhurst/infection-prevention

for example, age, diseases such as diabetes or cystic fibrosis, or infections such as human immunodeficiency virus (HIV). These are called *opportunistic pathogens* and a dental clinician must take particular care when taking a patient's medical history to enquire about conditions or drugs which may compromise the patient's immunity and make them more susceptible to infection. Steps should be taken to protect these vulnerable patients.

Breaking the chain of infection

A successful micro-organizm that can cause disease (a *pathogen*) must have a means of transmission from host to host, otherwise it would eventually disappear. The dental clinic is an environment where there are inherent infection risks which, unless they are controlled, offer the potential for pathogens to be transmitted from person to person. In order to cause disease rather than just superficial colonization, pathogens usually need a susceptible host, virulence factors to survive the challenges of the host immune system, and means of entering and exiting the body. Figure 2.1 illustrates the six components in the 'chain of infection' that lead eventually to disease. Links in the chain can be broken, halting further transmission and preventing disease. This positive outcome can be achieved by a combination of measures. Vaccination and drug therapy are used to protect the host, help eradicate the source and reservoir of the infection and treat the disease. Infection control and prevention measures can block the route of transmission and inhibit access to the portal of entry and exit, as depicted by the red crosses on Figure 2.1.

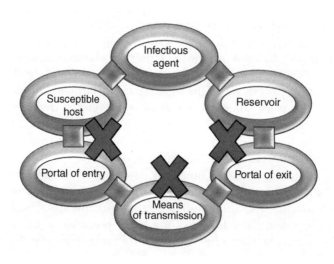

Figure 2.1 Breaking the chain of infection.

RESERVOIRS AND SOURCES OF INFECTION

A patient attending for dental treatment can act as a source of infection. In an outbreak situation they are referred to as the index case. He or she may present with one of the following four stages of infection/colonization.

- As a patient suffering from an acute infectious disease, for example influenza, measles, tuberculosis (TB).
- As a patient in the prodromal stage of infection, when the patient is infectious but not showing clinical symptoms, for example mumps or measles.
- As a patient in the convalescent or latent stage of infection, who continues to shed viruses in their secretions, for example herpes simplex virus (HSV), Ebola virus.
- As an asymptomatic carrier of potential pathogens, for example *Streptococcus pyogenes* (sore throat), methicillin-resistant *Staphylococcus aureus* (MRSA), *Neisseria meningitidis* (meningitis) and *Haemophilus influenzae* (bronchitis).

Patients with acute infection are usually very infectious and release large numbers of microbes into the environment. Those with serious infections rarely attend for routine clinical dentistry, but the dentist must be able and willing to treat such people if they require urgent care in a manner which will ensure the safety of themselves, other staff and patients, and is consistent with offering high standards of dental care to the patient. It is good policy to postpone elective dental treatment during the infective period, if it would improve the patient's comfort and eliminate the risk of cross-infection. Members of the dental team can also act as a source of infection, for example when they are suffering from an acute respiratory infection with a persistent cough or purulent skin infection, and should seek advice from their GP on their fitness to work.

Much attention has been focused on infectious asymptomatic carriers of hepatitis B virus (HBV) and hepatitis C virus (HCV) infection, as carriers may be unaware of their status and cannot be readily identified in the dental chair. Some patients may be aware of their carrier status but withhold information during medical history taking from fear of being refused treatment. Patients can be encouraged to reveal their carrier status by use of an empathic manner and appropriate questioning when taking their medical history. Asymptomatic carriers are often infective and HBV, HCV and HIV seropositive patients can represent some of the most serious risks for transmission of infection in dentistry. As we cannot reliably identify asymptomatic carriers, we apply the concept of universal precautions and manage *all* patients and their body fluids as if they were potentially infectious for a blood-borne virus (BBV) as part of the dental practice's Standard Infection Control Precautions (SICPs).

Healthcare-associated infections (HCAI), also referred to as nosocomial infections, are infections that are acquired or emerge during treatment or inpatient stay, and they are a major cause of concern to the medical and dental professions. In hospitals, infections are considered HCAI if they first appear 48 hours or more after hospital admission or within 30 days after discharge. Prevalence rates vary greatly but are of the order of 6–10% in many countries, with urinary tract infection and pneumonia the most prevalent. Outbreaks of MRSA, *Clostridium difficile* and antibiotic multiresistant organizms are a considerable cause of concern on hospital wards. Both in- and outpatients can become colonized with hospital-acquired multidrug-resistant organizms for considerable periods of time with the potential for spread in the community. The dental team must know how to prevent the spread of these microbes should such a patient present in their clinic. Prevention of spread can be achieved by simple infection control protocols such as hand hygiene and donning barriers for personal protection as discussed in Chapters 5 and 6.

INFECTIOUS DISEASES BY ROUTE OF INFECTION IN DENTISTRY

There are four main routes by which infection can be transmitted in a dental practice, as shown in Figure 2.2.

1. Transmission by direct or indirect contact, for example touching a surface with contaminated hands.
2. Percutaneous (parenteral) transmission, such as sharps injuries.
3. Transmission via air-borne route, for example aerosols generated by high-speed handpieces and respiratory secretions.
4. Common vehicle spread, such as dental unit waterlines and plumbing.

If you understand the route of transmission of an infective agent then you can choose the most effective measure to block cross-infection. Problems often arise when the routes of transmission of emerging infections pose a challenge to our existing methods for Standard Precautions. A good example is variant Creutzfeld–Jakob disease (vCJD) which is dealt with in greater depth in Chapter 7. Unlike most bacteria and viruses, vCJD is difficult to denature and remove from instruments by sterilization. Based on the results from experimental studies, our whole emphasis in the way we manage instrument sterilization in the UK had to change in response to the challenge posed by vCJD and prion diseases. Emerging infections force us to take a dynamic and inventive approach to infection control if we are not to be beaten by the microbes!

Globally, insect vectors such as mosquitoes are a major route of transmission of disease, including some of the most common and virulent disease known to humankind such as malaria, dengue, chikungunya, West Nile and Zika virus. Viruses spread by insects are known collectively as arboviruses and worldwide cause disease in hundreds of millions of people. Arboviruses can also be transmitted

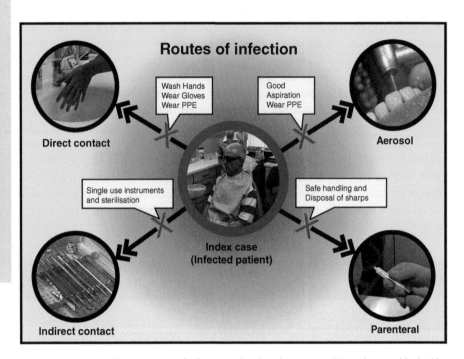

Figure 2.2 Routes of transmission of infection in the dental surgery and how they are blocked by standard infection control precautions. Source: Courtesy of Paul Morris.

by other modes of transmission. For example, Zika virus can cross the placenta, leading to Zika virus congenital syndrome and perinatal infection in newborns (e.g. microcephaly and other central nervous system abnormalities). Zika virus can be transmitted sexually in semen, which can result in cases of Zika virus infection occurring in partners of travellers returning home to areas of the world with a temperate climate that do not normally support mosquito transmission. Rarely, Zika virus has been reported to be transmitted during blood transfusions. Normally arboviruses would be expected to pose no greater threat to dentists or their patients above and beyond community exposure to bites from insect vectors.

INFECTIOUS DISEASE BY ROUTE OF TRANSMISSION IN THE DENTAL SURGERY

Direct and indirect contact spread of infection

Direct contact is the most easily appreciated mode of infection spread caused by dental professionals. Contact or direct spread occurs from person to person, or indirectly by touching surfaces contaminated by used equipment and splatter, or objects such as contaminated towels.

Pathogens transmitted by direct contact include the herpes group of viruses – herpes simplex virus (HSV), varicella zoster virus (VZV) and Epstein–Barr virus (EBV), HBV and viruses causing the common cold or flu. While we associate the spread of respiratory viruses mainly with aerosols generated during coughing, a hand politely placed in front of the mouth during a fit of coughing or holding a tissue to the nose when sneezing will become contaminated, as will every surface that hand touches. Hence the memorable slogan produced by the Department of Health in England: '*Catch it* (germs on a tissue), *bin it, kill it*' launched to help reduce the spread of flu in public places.

Herpes simplex virus is very infectious and yet patients do not hesitate to attend a dental clinic with herpes labialis (cold sore). Prior to the use of gloves in dentistry, dentists often picked up a second primary HSV through small abrasions on their fingers whilst treating a patient with a cold sore. Known as a herpetic whitlow, these intensely painful skin lesions can persist for several weeks and would prevent the person from working. Viral infections that across the placenta during pregnancy, such as VZV, which causes chickenpox and shingles, and rubella, pose a risk to the unborn fetus and pregnant women. In many countries, including the UK, dentists and clinical members of the dental team must be vaccinated against VZV and rubella infection if they have no natural immunity in order to prevent transmitting the infection to a pregnant woman.

Many bacterial infections could potentially be transmitted by direct and indirect contact in the dental clinic, but the one which causes most concern, especially in oral surgery, is *S. aureus*, in particular MRSA. The latter infection is defined by resistance to an old antibiotic, methicillin (meticillin), but it is important because MRSA demonstrates resistant to most types of penicillin and cephalosporins. About 25–30% of the population are colonized with *S. aureus,* but MRSA is only carried by approximately 1–3% of people, more if they have recently been in a hospital or other healthcare facility (including residential homes) where MRSA is endemic. The main mode of transmission of MRSA is via the hands of the HCW, which may become contaminated by direct contact either from colonized or infected patients or objects (fomites) in the immediate environment surrounding the patient. Dentists who provide a locum service to patients in a residential home should ensure that they are rigorous in their hand hygiene and use of PPE in order to reduce their risk of becoming colonized with MRSA.

Panton-Valentine Leukocidin (PVL) *S. aureus* infection infects mainly younger populations in the community and can, if left untreated, cause very severe skin infections and, more rarely, lung abscesses. Primarily, the infection affects athletes, children attending daycare centres and intravenous drug users, situations where there is close skin-to-skin contact and spread is encouraged by poor hygiene. Once again, unless the dental team practises good hand hygiene and contact precautions are applied, they are at risk of occupational infection.

COMMUNICABLE DISEASES IN THE DENTAL SURGERY

Prevention of person-to-person spread of infection

The primary source of spread from person to person is by hands and clothing and this route of infection is easily interrupted by hand washing and wearing of gloves and disposable aprons (see Figure 2.1), as outlined in Chapter 5.

Prevention of indirect spread of infection from equipment

Equipment including dental instruments must be decontaminated between patients (see Figure 2.2) or be discarded safely if they are designated single use, as outlined in Chapter 7. Dental impressions should be disinfected to reduce the risk of infection to dental technicians and comply with regulations concerning the transport of infected material by postal services. Dental chairs and units must also be cleaned and disinfected between patients and this is facilitated by dividing the surgery into 'zones' of different levels of contamination, as outlined in Chapter 8.

Prevention of spread of infection by fluids

The dental unit waterlines are a potential source of the spread of infection by both aerosol and indirect contact, and the management and methods of reducing these risks are discussed in Chapter 9. Disinfectant and detergents must be stored in concentrated form according to the manufacturer's recommendation as they can become a source of infection by bacteria such as *Pseudomonas aeruginosa* which can be resistant to some disinfectants and pose a risk to immunocompromised patients.

The transmission of infection via food is a major source of concern in society but should not be a risk in dentistry, since no food should be taken in surgery and adequate kitchen facilities should be provided for staff.

Percutaneous transmission of infection

Many organizms are potentially transmissible in the occupational setting via percutaneous (sharps) (see Figure 2.2) or mucocutaneous (mucous membrane/broken skin) routes. The so-called *blood-borne viruses* (BBVs) are our primary concern. The BBVs, which present the most significant cross-infection hazard to HCWs, are those that exhibit carrier states with persistent viraemia and replication. These include HIV and hepatitis B and C.

Hepatitis B virus

Hepatitis B is blood borne and sexually transmitted. The virus is a member of the Hepadnaviridae DNA family, which causes inflammation of the liver. The incubation period is 45–160 days (average 120 days). In areas of the world where the prevalence of HBV is high (greater than 2% of the population are seropositive for hepatitis B surface antigen (HBsAg)), transmission is mostly perinatal or during childhood through horizontal transmission from close household contacts. In low-prevalence countries such as North America and in parts of Europe, transmission usually occurs later in life during heterosexual and homosexual sexual intercourse with an infected partner or by intravenous drug misuse. The natural history of HBV infection is influenced by the age at which an individual is infected. Neonatal infections are generally asymptomatic, but in most cases lead to chronic infection (90%) whereas infection in adults is more likely to result in symptomatic acute hepatitis, but with a lower risk of persistent infection (5–10%). Many acutely infected adults have no obvious symptoms, but 30–50% experience fatigue, fever, loss of appetite with nausea, vomiting, abdominal discomfort, joint pain and jaundice. The vast majority of those with acute disease recover with no lasting liver damage and the acute illness is rarely fatal. In contrast, 15–25% of chronically infected people develop chronic liver disease, including cirrhosis, liver failure or liver cancer. The persistence of the 'e' antigen and high HBV-DNA levels correlate with a high level of viral replication and increased infectivity. Hepatitis B infection persisting for longer than six months is defined as a chronic infection.

According to the WHO, a third of the world's population has been infected with HBV, with an estimated 14 million people chronically infected in the WHO European region. Hepatitis B vaccine can prevent hepatitis B infection. Since 1991, the WHO has recommended universal hepatitis B vaccination of all newborns and children up to 18 years, as well as vaccination of at-risk groups. The incidence of the disease has decreased significantly in countries that have implemented this policy. Vaccination has played a key role in prevention of HBV infection within the dental profession and is part of SICP policy. It is, however, not a substitute for the safe practices outlined in Chapter 3. Currently, HCV and HIV pose a risk of infection which cannot be mitigated by prophylactic vaccination.

Hepatitis C virus

Hepatitis C virus causes both acute and chronic infection of the liver. Acute HCV infection is usually asymptomatic, and is only very rarely associated with life-threatening disease. About 15–45% of infected persons spontaneously clear the virus within six months of infection without any treatment. The remaining 55–85% will develop chronic HCV infection, many of whom are unaware of their infection. In patients with chronic HCV infection, 15–30% are diagnosed with cirrhosis of the liver within 20 years of their initial infection, of whom 20% will develop liver cancer.

The global burden of people chronically infected with HCV is estimated at 130–150 million. High levels of endemic infection are reported in Africa and Central and East Asia. In the UK, HCV chronic infection has increased by a third over the last decade, with approximately 214 000 people living with chronic HCV. Most HCV infections arise from needle sharing by people injecting recreational, performance and image-enhancing drugs or medical and dental unsafe injection practices. The first proven case of HCV transmission from patient to patient in a dental office happened recently in Tulsa, USA, during patient treatment under IV sedation. The dental staff habitually used the same needle to give both the initial dose of IV sedation drug and any additional top-up drug that was required during sedation treatment. Any residual IV sedation drug remaining in the drug vial was then used to sedate the next patient. Unfortunately for the index case, the reused drug vial on this occasion was previously used on an HCV seropositive patient who had required multiple drug doses to achieve sedation. Scientists from the CDC, Atlanta, were able to demonstrate conclusively with the aid of molecular genetic techniques that HCV was transmitted as a direct consequence of the staff reusing an HCV infected single-use drug vial.

HIV transmission

The most common modes of HIV transmission include unprotected oral and penetrative sexual intercourse, and sharing of needles and syringes when injecting drugs. Due to the benefits of effective treatment and prevention measures, once common routes of transmission such as mother-to-child transmission and transfusion of HIV-contaminated blood or blood products are greatly reduced. In the dental clinic, prevention focuses on safe handling and disposal of sharp instruments and training of staff. Even though the risk of infection with HIV is 100 times less than HBV for a similar exposure, the stigma and fear of the consequences of infection have often shaken dentists' confidence in their infection control measures, to the extent that HIV seropositive patients have in the past experienced difficulty obtaining dental treatment. Fortunately, as a result of several initiatives the situation has now changed radically. HIV-infected HCWs are permitted to work as dentists/therapists/hygienists in most countries of the world, including the UK (see Chapter 3), and effective postexposure prophylaxis drugs are available following a exposure incident (see Chapter 4).

The recommended approach internationally is to encourage routine screening for HIV in healthcare settings and targeted screening of at-risk groups in non-healthcare settings. If a person remains undiagnosed, they cannot benefit from advances in drug treatments that reduce viral load and increase their immune function and life expectancy. Furthermore, they are unlikely to continue to infect others if they have an undetectable viral load. Studies show that early use of combination antiretroviral therapy (cART) before the immune system is compromised results in better clinical outcomes for people living with HIV. Daily oral pre-exposure prophylaxis (PrEP) drugs are now recommended for people at substantial risk of HIV infection, for example the partners of HIV-infected patients, as part of a combination prevention approach. The UK is one of many countries succeeding in meeting the United Nations'ambitious sustainable development goal, which sets a global target of ≥90% of persons living with HIV knowing their serostatus, ≥90% of persons living with diagnosed HIV infection receiving ART and ≥90% of persons receiving ART having viral suppression, by 2020. For those of us working in dentistry, the UNAIDS '90:90:90' goals will in the future eliminate the risks associated with the provision of dental treatment for HIV patients. However, there is no room for complacency at the current time. It is important that an individual dental HCW or student is confident that the practice's or dental school's standard infection control measures are sufficient to reduce the risk of transmission of HIV and other BBVs to negligible levels. The prevention of BBV infection in dentistry is the subject of Chapter 3.

Spread of infection by air-borne and respiratory secretions

Dental personnel are exposed to aerosolized water from the dental unit waterlines as well as aerosols of the patient's saliva, blood and respiratory secretions, generated during use of high-speed rotary instruments and ultrasonic scalers. The risk of occupational infection from waterlines is mainly from legionellae and the management of waterlines is considered in Chapter 9.

Organizms which may be transmitted in aerosols include *Mycobacterium tuberculosis* and respiratory viruses, such as rhinoviruses (cause the common cold), adenoviruses and influenza viruses. Some of the herpes viruses such as VZV and EBV can also be transmitted from respiratory secretions.

Tuberculosis

Tuberculosis ranks alongside HIV/AIDS as a leading cause of death worldwide. Many patients globally are co-infected with TB and HIV, requiring active treatment of both diseases. Ending the global TB epidemic is one of the WHO's sustainable development goals. Massive improvements have occurred globally. Reported TB prevalence in 2015 was 42% lower than in 1990, with a success rate for treatment of new infections of 86%. Since the majority of cases are in resource-poor countries, many dentists do not perceive TB to be a risk in their practice, even though certain metropolitan areas of England have the highest number of TB cases in Western Europe, with a prevalence of infection five times that of the USA. The reason for the high prevalence of TB is social factors such as urban homelessness, history of imprisonment, intravenous drug or alcohol abuse, recurrence in the elderly and migration of populations from areas of high incidence. Multidrug-resistant TB is a great cause of concern globally and accounts for an estimated 3.3% of new TB cases and 20% of previously treated cases.

Transmission of infection from dentist to patient is rare. However, there was a report of an outbreak of TB affecting tooth sockets that occurred in 15 child patients following dental extractions by a community dentist with active TB in 1982. This potential risk of infection transmission is the reason the UK recommends that all new HCWs be assessed regarding personal or family history of TB. BCG vaccination should be offered to HCWs, irrespective of age, who:

- are previously unvaccinated (that is, without adequate documentation or a characteristic scar), and
- will have contact with patients or clinical materials, and
- are Mantoux skin test negative (or test positive with an interferon-gamma release assay for latent TB).

The prevention of aerosol and splatter transmission involves the application of standard precautions with emphasis on having a well-ventilated surgery (up to 12–15 air changes per hour), the control of aerosols by high-volume suction, externally ventilated aspiration, and wearing of surgical or respirator masks, goggles and visors for personal protection, and use of a rubber dam as discussed in Chapters 6 and 8.

Influenza

Influenza virus causes a respiratory illness with the symptoms of headache, fever, coryza, cough, sore throat, aching muscles and joints and sometimes gastrointestinal symptoms. Each year, approximately 10% of Europe's population is infected. Influenza-related complications (such as lower respiratory tract infection, central nervous system involvement and/or a significant exacerbation of an underlying medical condition) cause hundreds of thousands of hospitalizations across Europe.

The incubation period of human influenza ranges from one to four days (typically 2–3). Infectivity is proportional to symptom severity and maximal just after the onset of symptoms, and the period of communicability is typically up to five days after symptom onset in adults and seven days in children, but can be considerably prolonged in immunocompromised patients. There are two main types of influenza virus, with type A usually causing more severe symptoms than type B.

Because flu usually occurs every winter in the UK, it is referred to as *seasonal flu* and must be differentiated from *pandemic flu* and *avian flu*, which can occur at any time of year. Control of influenza outbreaks worldwide relies on a three-pronged approach:

- annual vaccination of susceptible groups and HCWs

- targeted treatment/prophylaxis with influenza antiviral neuraminidase inhibitors (antivirals), for example oseltamivir and zanamivir
- hand hygiene and respiratory etiquette (see Chapters 3, 5 and 6).

It is advised that dental professionals with flu-like symptoms and/or fever should not work with patients and colleagues. Health protection authorities in European countries, and globally via the WHO, monitor and record the incidence of seasonal flu strains and the uptake of seasonal flu vaccine. This information is used to guide the choice of viral strains incorporated within the annual seasonal flu vaccine, as well as development of policies for protecting the population from influenza. These organizations alert health professionals, including dentists, if there is increased incidence of flu. HCWs are strongly encouraged to be vaccinated against seasonal flu annually.

Influenza viruses are spread in the respiratory secretions which are generated by coughing or sneezing. Transmission is by direct contact on hands and indirect contact by large respiratory droplets contaminating surfaces which are then touched. Influenza viruses can survive on environmental surfaces such as glass or plastic and be transferred to hands for up to 24 hours. On porous materials such as clothing, magazines and tissues, the virus can survive for 2–4 hours. Influenza viruses are easily deactivated by washing hands with soap and water or alcohol-based hand sanitizers and cleaning surfaces with household detergents.

Pandemic influenza and avian flu

Pandemics arise when a new virus emerges which is capable of crossing international boundaries and infecting large numbers of people worldwide. This was the situation during the influenza pandemic of 1918–19, when a completely new influenza virus subtype (influenza A/H1N1) emerged and spread around the globe in waves over a two-year period, killing an estimated 40–50 million people. Pandemics can have such a devastating impact as most of the population is non-immune to the new virus, except some of the elderly who may have experienced a similar virus previously. There have been three subsequent influenza pandemics, in 1957–8, 1968–9 and 2009–10. There are continuing concerns that circulating avian influenza virus strains or novel reassortments of human with animal (swine) and/or bird flu virus strains may give rise to the next pandemic influenza virus.

The precautions required in the event of an outbreak of pandemic or avian flu are similar to those for seasonal flu described above. The only difference is that there is a national contingency plan for the outbreak, and HCWs will be instructed when to present for vaccination and acquisition of prophylactic antiviral drugs, as occurred in 2010. Strict adherence to standard infection control practice, in particular PPE and hand washing, is essential (see Chapters 5 and 6).

EMERGING AND RE-EMERGING PATHOGENS

Emerging and re-emerging infections are diseases that are reported in a population for the first time, or that may have existed previously but are rapidly increasing in incidence or geographic range. Infections can emerge via a variety of different processes.

- Novel pathogens arising *de novo* due to genetic mutations or evolution of existing human or animal infections, for example pandemic influenza, vCJD, MERS.
- Known infections spreading to new geographic areas or populations, such as West Nile virus in the USA, Ebola in West Africa, Zika virus into Central and South America.
- Previously unreported infections appearing in areas undergoing climate change, such as chikungunya and dengue.
- Old infections re-emerging as a result of changes in host immunity, antimicrobial selection and resistance or breakdowns in public health measures such as national vaccination campaigns, for example polio, syphilis, diphtheria and MDR-TB.

Infections tend to become more prevalent when conditions allow for their transmission and may recede into the background over time as the conditions change. Recent examples include Ebola virus disease in West African in 2013–15 and pandemic influenza outbreaks in 2010.

Why do infections emerge?

Rapid globalization, changes in climate and global warming, agricultural practices, urbanization, antibiotic selection and health status of the population (immunosuppression or famine) can all facilitate emergence of disease. Worldwide, mosquitoes and other insect vectors constitute a major mode of transmission of blood-borne viral infections such as dengue, chikungunya, Zika and West Nile virus infections. Global warming has permitted disease-carrying species of mosquitoes to survive in more northerly countries in Europe and traditionally tropical diseases such as dengue and chikungunya have been transmitted by mosquitoes in France and Italy. Even in the UK, scientists have predicted that by 2030–50, increases in summer temperature in southern England will be enough for malaria-carrying mosquitoes to thrive.

Increased access to travel and migration of people have a strong association with the spread of infection. The Black Death in the Middle Ages was associated with increased travel by ships and new risks are posed by increased travel by air. In 2013, 842 million people travelled by air in the European Union, and 39% of these flights were to countries outside the European Union. This is the reason why information on recent travel outside the country of origin is important for identifying emerging infections as the patient may have contracted the infection abroad and only develop symptoms upon returning home.

The impact of emerging infections on dentistry

Emerging pathogens are of importance in the dentistry for two reasons. First, they challenge our infection control and prevention protocols and prompt the question 'Is there a risk of transmission of this particular infection in the dental surgery?'. Second, 'novel infections' can shake the confidence of the public and the dental team and therefore we need to educate ourselves regarding such disease so that we can perform appropriate risk assessments and reassure ourselves and the public that dental treatment is safe.

Zoonosis and the evolution of novel infections

Some microbes such as avian influenza virus, rabies virus, Ebola virus, Middle Eastern respiratory virus (MERS) and *Salmonella* use wild or domestic animals as their primary host and occasionally infect humans (incidental host). Transmission from animal to humans occurs through a number of different routes, including direct contact with the living animal, their meat and secretions or vector transmission via insect bites. These are known as *zoonotic* infections and are important in the evolution of novel infections affecting human populations. Emerging zoonotic infections can pose a significant risk to human populations, for example avian flu, as there may be no or limited natural immunity to these novel infections.

Zoonoses occur in farm animals such as cattle. An example was bovine spongiform encephalitis (BSE, mad cow disease) that jumped species to cause vCJD in humans and was eventually controlled by culling the primary host, young calves. But when the zoonosis has its reservoir in a wild forest animal such as the fruit bat, as occurred with the largest ever human outbreak of Ebola virus disease in West Africa (2013–15), then mass culling of a wild animal is not an option. During the initial stages of the Ebola outbreak, drug treatments and anti-Ebola vaccines were in the experimental trial stage of development and were only available for use late in the outbreak. Therefore, the Ebola outbreak was eventually brought under control by a concerted national and international campaign that relied on well-tried measures from the pre-antimicrobial era. These included public education, contact tracing and quarantine of suspected cases, local curfews, border controls, modification of burial practices and, most importantly, rigorous infection control and prevention measures.

Operative dentistry could potentially offer a secondary route for person-to-person transmission of zoonotic infections that are transmitted by direct contact, respiratory and percutaneous routes. Let us look at two examples of emerging zoonotic infections that have had an impact on the dental profession.

Novel coronavirus infections

SARS-CoV and MERS-CoV are caused by coronaviruses in the same family as the common cold virus but they cause a severe acute respiratory illness. SARS emerged in China in 2003 and resulted in 8437 probable cases with 813 deaths. SARS was successfully eradicated and useful lessons were learnt from the management of that outbreak, such as the correct order in which to remove PPE (see Chapter 6). A decade later, a new coronavirus emerged in the Middle East, called MERS-CoV.

What alarmed the world community about SARS was its rate of spread and it was termed a *superspreader* as it spread rapidly around the world from China to Canada. The virus had multiple sites of replication in the body and was spread during close contact via respiratory secretions and faeces. Infectivity increased as the disease progressed and reached a maximum around day 10 when the patient was very seriously ill. This is the reason why about one-third of cases occurred in HCWs. A similar pattern is seen with MERS transmission. The initial epidemiological picture was consistent with sporadic zoonotic infections from human contact with camel secretions and meat, with amplification of the spread of infection within healthcare premises during patient treatment. Onward transmission is now mainly from person to person.

Outbreaks of MERS are associated with delays in identification of cases, multiple contacts within healthcare and gaps in infection control protocols. Typically, the large outbreak in South Korea in 2015 arose from an imported index case – a doctor from the Middle East. At the end of the outbreak, 186 people had developed MERS, of whom 36 died. All these cases, with the exception of the index case, were linked to a single chain of transmission associated with the hospital where he was treated. A salutary lesson for those of us working in dentistry is that during the SARS outbreak in 2003, the decision was made to close the dental school in Hong Kong for many months as a public health measure. This step was taken in order to protect the general public, staff and dental students from any additional exposure to SARS, arising as a direct consequence of the enhanced risk of respiratory transmission from dental aerosols.

Variant Creutzfeldt–Jakob disease and transmissible spongiform encephalopathy agents

Human cases of vCJD linked to consuming beef tainted with BSE were first diagnosed in 1995. vCJD cases peaked in 2000, with six deaths per quarter in mid-2000 with a declining incidence recorded since. The total number of deaths from vCJD worldwide is approximately 229, the majority of whom (178 cases; figures up to April 2016) were in the UK. In contrast to HIV, TB and pandemic flu, vCJD has killed very few people and has not spread rapidly around the globe, yet this disease has had a major impact on how we practise dentistry, particularly in the UK, and has raised awareness of prion disease internationally.

vCJD is not caused by a living entity containing a genetic code for its reproduction; rather, the disease is caused by a 'rogue protein' molecule called a *prion*, which belongs to a group of diseases known as transmissible spongiform encephalopathies (TSE). While CJD prions are confined to the central nervous system (CNS), vCJD prions are detected in the CNS and in the peripheral nervous system and lymphoid tissues. Four cases of transmission of vCJD, three via blood transfusion and one from plasma-derived products, were reported in 2003–4 in the UK. Each of the cases had received blood from donors who appeared well at the time of donation, but later died of vCJD. Fortunately, blood does not appear to be an efficient vehicle for transmission of vCJD. Prions have also been identified in the trigeminal ganglion and tonsils from vCJD patients at postmortem. Dental pulp, which is composed of vascular and peripheral nerve tissue, was shown to be infected with vCJD in animal studies.

There is evidence to support a carrier state for vCJD. This data is based on the testing of 12 000 tonsils plus 32 000 appendices from 41 hospitals removed surgically from 2000 to 2012. The extrapolated figures indicate that approximately one in 2000 people in the UK may be a carrier of vCJD. In addition, over 6350 patients in the UK are thought to have been potentially exposed to vCJD or CJD through surgical instruments, dura mater grafts, human-derived growth hormones or blood/pooled plasma transfusions (iatrogenic exposure). These patients pose a small but significant public health risk as tissue, organ or blood products or inadequately decontaminated instruments used on such patients could potentially transmit vCJD or CJD (see Chapter 7 for management). These patients are notified of the public health risk they pose and are monitored long term. To identify such patients, dentists are advised to include the following question on medical history and consent forms:

> Have you ever been notified that you are at increased risk of CJD or vCJD for public health purposes?

How many of these patients will develop disease in the future is unknown. As with all emerging pathogens, our knowledge base continues to evolve as our understanding grows. Therefore, as a precaution, at-risk patients are advised not to donate blood, other tissues or organs. They are requested to inform their medical and dental carers prior to any invasive procedures, such as removal of third molars or oral surgery procedures involving cranial nerves or tonsillar tissue. If invasive treatment is required then the patient should be managed in secondary care as the instruments used on the patient may require quarantine or disposal according to latest guidance issued by the Advisory Committee on Dangerous Pathogens – Transmissible Spongiform Encephalopathy Working Group.

A patient with, or 'at increased risk' of, CJD or vCJD should not be refused routine dental treatment. Such people can be treated in the same way as any member of the general public and instruments used on them can be decontaminated safely using the methods described in Chapter 7. NHS England stated in HTM 01-05 that 'the risk of transmission from dental instruments is very low provided optimal standards of infection control and decontamination are maintained'. This has been the source of much debate as the definition of 'optimal decontamination standards' can vary greatly between countries. To this end, the CJD International Surveillance Unit is collecting data to identify secondary routes of transmission of vCJD, including, amongst others, dentistry. Much of the guidance outlined in this book in relation to instrument decontamination and the increased use of single-use instruments has been with the stated aim of improving decontamination processes to a level that instruments used on patients who may be unknown carriers vCJD can be safely reused on other patients. Routine sterilization at 134 °C does not guarantee complete inactivation of prions. Therefore, the emphasis has shifted to highly effective presterilization washing and rinsing of instruments to remove and destroy prion protein prior to sterilization. Improvements in standards that have been introduced in instrument decontamination, sterilization and periodic testing are discussed further in Chapter 7.

The bottom line is that no matter what new or emerging infections arise in the future, so long as there is accurate information regarding their routes of transmission, the dental team can remain resilient to the challenge. We can make use of the deceptively simple dual concepts of chain of infection and standard precautions to modify our infection control protocols in dentistry to cope with any new situation. We live in a dynamic world and the topics outlined in this book should make you better able to meet changes in the future.

REFERENCES AND WEBSITES

Gill ON, Richard-Loendt A, Kelly C *et al.* (2013) Prevalent abnormal prion protein in human appendixes after bovine spongiform encephalopathy epizootic: large scale survey. *British Medical Journal*, **347**, f5675.

Klevens RM, Gorwitz RJ, Collins AS. (2008) Methicillin-resistant Staphylococcus aureus. A primer for dentists. *Journal of the American Dental Association*, **139**, 1328–1337.

Medlock JM, Leach SA. (2015) Effect of climate change on vector-borne disease risk in the UK. *Lancet Infectious Diseases*, **15**, 721–730.

Oklahoma State Department of Health (2013) Dental Healthcare-Associated Transmission of Hepatitis C. Final Report of Public Health Investigation and Response. Available at: www.ok.gov/health2/documents/Dental%20Healthcare_Final%20Report_2_17_15.pdf (accessed 27 October 2016).

Smales FC, Samaranyake LP. (2003) Maintaining dental education and specialist dental care during an outbreak of a new coronavirus infection. Part 1: A deadly viral epidemic begins. *British Dental Journal*, **195**, 557–561.

Chapter 3

Occupational health and immunization

OCCUPATIONAL HEALTH HAZARDS

In the working environment, members of the dental team are exposed to a variety of hazardous substances as well as microbial pathogens. If you want to stay healthy in the dental practice then the first step is to identify where the major infection-associated occupational health hazards might lie.

- Sharps injuries and exposure to blood-borne virus (see Chapter 4)
- Respiratory infections from inhaling contaminated aerosols generated from the dental unit waterlines, e.g. Legionnaires' disease, Pontiac fever (see Chapter 9)
- Exposure to respiratory aerosols from infected patients, e.g. tuberculosis (TB), influenza (see Chapter 2)
- Eye and skin infections, e.g. herpetic whitlow, impetigo, conjunctivitis (see Chapter 2)
- Hypersensitive reactions affecting skin and respiratory system, e.g. natural rubber latex (see Chapter 6)
- Mercury toxicity (see Chapter 10)

Health and safety law requires the employer to implement measures to protect all members of the dental team from such hazards as far as is reasonably practicable.

Basic Guide to Infection Prevention and Control in Dentistry, Second Edition.
Caroline L. Pankhurst.
© 2017 John Wiley & Sons Ltd. Published 2017 by John Wiley & Sons Ltd.
Companion website: www.wiley.com/go/pankhurst/infection-prevention

BUILDING A CULTURE OF SAFETY

One of the main strategies for combating transmission of infection from person to person within the practice is to develop a culture of safety. Safe working practices, compliance with infection control policies, reporting injuries and near misses and effective management form the backbone of a dental practice's safety culture. Personal protective equipment (PPE) (see Chapter 6), sharps incorporating safety devices, immunization and postexposure prophylaxis (see Chapter 5) all contribute to the protective 'defences' against transmission of infection. Figure 3.1 illustrates how all these factors could come together to create a culture of safety within the dental practice.

This approach requires a commitment from the whole dental team if it is to be successful. Everyone in the dental team, including students and trainees, has an important contribution to make. Some of the steps the dental practice can take to create a safety culture are shown in Box 3.1. As part of the induction process and ongoing training, members of the team are normally asked to read and sign the practice's current infection control policy.

Accidents such as sharps injuries will occur in the practice, however well it is run, but it is important to try and understand why an accident or a near miss occurred to prevent it from happening again. Mistakes and accidents tend not to be random mishaps but to fall into recurrent patterns, referred to as *error traps*. The same set of circumstances can provoke similar errors or accidents regardless

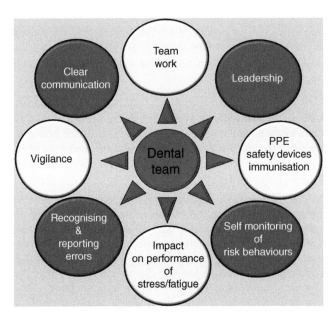

Figure 3.1 How the dental team can work together to build a safety culture.

Box 3.1   Steps involved in creating a practice safety culture

A safety culture is created through:
- actions the practice management takes to improve patient and dental personnel safety
- all the members of the dental team participating in safety planning and infection control protocol development
- influence of group norms regarding acceptable safety practices
- routine and occupational immunization, postexposure prophylaxis, availability of appropriate personal protective equipment and training in its correct use
- induction training and socialization process for new dental personnel or students

---

of the member of staff or student involved. To be effective, cross-infection prevention necessitates looking beyond the simple explanation that it was someone's fault and attempting to answer the much harder question as to why the error occurred in the first place. There is seldom a single reason. Breakdowns in the practice's infection control management and 'defences' can arise from two main causes:

- active failures
- latent conditions.

Active failures are unsafe acts committed by frontline people in direct contact with the patient. Their impact is usually instantaneous and breaches the integrity of the practice's 'defences'. In many cases, unsafe acts have a causal history that extends back in time. The case scenario example given below shows how active and latent failures can combine and stack up with serious long-term consequences.

Example of an active failure: During a surgical extraction on a patient with hepatitis B, the suture needle is covered by a bloody swab and both are discarded into a waste sack. The needle punctures the waste sack and the cleaner receives a sharps injury when she empties the pedal bin.

Example of a series of latent failure: A temporary cleaner from an agency was covering for the practice's regular cleaner who was on holiday. She had not been vaccinated against hepatitis B (which is a requirement for all people who come into contact with body fluids or hazardous clinical waste as part of their job). No one at the agency or the dental practice had checked if she was vaccinated against hepatitis B. Three months later she was diagnosed with hepatitis B. She worked at night after the practice had closed and had not reported the accident. As there was no record of the incident in the accident book, she was unable to prove how and where she acquired the infection and was unable to make an insurance claim to which she would have been entitled.

┌───┐
│ **Box 3.2   Where latent failures could occur in dental practice** │
├───┤
│ Poor design of surgery and equipment   │
│ Ineffective training   │
│ Inadequate supervision   │
│ Ineffective communications   │
│ Uncertainties in roles and responsibilities   │
└───┘

Latent failures arise from decisions made on the design, procedures and management within the practice (Box 3.2) or may relate to decisions taken outside the dental practice by third parties, such as equipment and instrument manufacturers or governmental organizations. Latent or delayed failures can remain dormant for many years until they combine with active failures and other local triggers to create an opportunity for an accident. If the dental practice's infection control policy and 'defences' function as intended, the results of the unsafe act are caught and the effects limited. If not, the accident could have tragic and long-term consequences (as in the examples above). To prevent latent failures causing repeated incidents, they require proactive rather than reactive responses from the dental team.

A way of highlighting active and latent failures in the dental practice is to use root cause analysis. Staff and students working on the 'frontline' are usually in the best position to identify issues and solution. The aim of a root cause analysis is to determine:

- what happened
- why it happened
- what can be done to prevent it from happening again.

ORGANIZING STAFF HEALTH IN A DENTAL PRACTICE

Everyone working in the practice has a duty of care towards the patients, which includes taking reasonable precautions to protect them from communicable diseases. This can be achieved by appropriate immunization against vaccine-preventable diseases. But immunization should never be regarded as a substitute for safe working. Immunization directly protects the individual, and indirectly protects their family and friends, colleagues and vulnerable patients. Preventing common communicable infections such as influenza promotes efficient running of the dental practice and reduces disruptions caused by sick leave.

Immunization policy and staff health records

Dentists as employers are required to demonstrate that they have an effective employee immunization policy in place based on national guidance, for example 'Immunization against infectious disease' (The Green Book). It is normally recommended that the practice nominates a person to co-ordinate the administration of staff health and the reporting and recording of accidents and near misses within the practice. The practice should keep a confidential record of health clearance records, including hepatitis B antibody test results and occupational immunization schedules. Inclusion of an alerting system helps ensure that the records are contemporary and that all members of the dental team are up to date with booster vaccinations. Pre-employment health clearance, evaluation of immunization status and eligibility for vaccinations according to the national schedule are normally managed by an occupational health service provider. They can also advise on circumstances under which staff may need to be excluded from work and provide assessment of sharps and splash incidents.

Failure to report accidents

Recent data suggest that 35% of dentists failed to report sharps injuries even though there is a legal requirement to do so. Underreporting of sharps and splash incidents is a common phenomenon in healthcare. It is helpful if the occupational health co-ordinator in the dental practice understands the reasons why injuries are not reported and addresses barriers to reporting that apply in their own practice.

Failure to report accidents, incidences or near misses is often due to:

- fear of being accused of negligence
- fear of being labelled accident prone
- damage to reputation with peers
- conflict of loyalty to the patient or the practice
- fear of subsequent medical treatment, e.g. postexposure prophylaxis
- fear of exclusion from work
- lack of understanding of purpose of accident reporting.

A wise man (the poet Alexander Pope) said, 'To err is human, to forgive, divine'. High-risk industries with the potential for disastrous accidents such as aviation and nuclear power are pioneers in the field of industrial safety. Their good safety record is based on a non-blame approach, with the emphasis firmly on prevention, not punishment. Both industries have found this to be the best method to encourage reporting of incidents and near misses by their staff.

IMMUNIZATION REQUIREMENTS FOR DENTISTRY

In the UK, it is recommended that all clinical and non-clinical healthcare workers, trainees and students are up to date with routine vaccinations against tetanus, diphtheria, polio and measles, mumps and rubella (MMR). All dental healthcare workers and students who have close contact with patients will require additional BCG immunization that protects against TB. BCG vaccine is not routinely recommended for non-clinical staff in healthcare settings. Varicella vaccine is recommended for all susceptible (non-immune) members of the dental team, including receptionists, who have close or regular patient contact but are not necessarily involved in direct patient care. All staff members in the dental practice and students who are exposed to blood or blood-stained body fluids or are at risk of sharps injury or of being deliberately bitten or injured by patients should be vaccinated against hepatitis B, including cleaning staff and receptionists (Table 3.1). Annual vaccination against seasonal influenza is strongly recommended for all members of the dental team and students directly involved in patient care. Influenza vaccination is not routinely recommended for non-clinical staff members.

PROTECTING WOMEN OF CHILDBEARING AGE

Women of childbearing age working in the dental practice should protect themselves from occupational infections that can cause damage to the fetus during pregnancy, e.g. rubella, varicella and syphilis.

MMR vaccine

Mumps, measles and rubella vaccine is recommended as an occupational vaccine for healthcare workers. During the first decade of the twenty-first century a distrust of the MMR vaccine developed amongst parents that led to a poor uptake of the vaccine in the UK. This misunderstanding was fuelled by adverse publicity surrounding an unsubstantiated and later discredited claim of an association between MMR vaccination and an increased risk of autism in children. Low vaccine uptake resulted in a resurgence of mumps and measles with outbreaks of infection reported throughout the UK and then in continental Europe. This fall in herd immunity left a cohort of adults born between 1980 and 1995 at risk of infection who were too old to receive the MMR vaccine when it was first introduced, and had not developed natural immunity. Healthcare workers who are non-immune to rubella and measles on serological testing are recommended to receive two doses of MMR vaccine (see Table 3.1).

Table 3.1 Recommended occupational immunization

Disease	Occupational route of spread	Pre- or postimmunization serological testing	Type of vaccine	Dosing schedule in healthcare workers	Occupational immunization recommendation
Varicella (chickenpox, shingles)	Respiratory droplets or direct contact with blisters, contaminated clothing	Pretesting	Varicella live attenuated vaccine	Two doses 4–8 weeks apart	All non-immune dental workers who have direct or regular patient contact
Tuberculosis	Respiratory droplets	Pretesting; Mantoux test; (interferon-gamma release assay)	BCG; live attenuated, derived from *Mycobacterium bovis*	Single dose	Dental workers with close patient contact (unvaccinated, tuberculin-negative individuals)
Hepatitis B	Sharps injuries and blood exposure of mucous membranes or non-intact skin	Post immunization	Inactivated	Three or four doses; reinforcing vaccination at 5 years or as prophylaxis following sharps/mucosal injury	All staff who have contact with blood or blood-stained body fluids or risk of sharps injury with no evidence of previous immunization or disease
Mumps, measles, rubella (MMR)	Droplet spread	N/A	Live attenuated	Two doses	All dental workers unless documented evidence of two doses of MMR, or positive antibody tests for measles and rubella
Influenza	Aerosols, droplets and direct contact	N/A	Trivalent, containing two subtypes of influenza A and one type B virus	Single dose	All dental workers directly involved in patient care

Rubella

Rubella is a mild disease caused by a togavirus; it is spread by droplet transmission. It may begin with a prodromal illness involving a low-grade fever, malaise and mild conjunctivitis. The erythematous (red) rubella rash on the ears, face and neck can easily be missed as it is transitory. Incubation period is 14–21 days, and the person is infectious from one week before symptoms appear to four days after the onset of the rash. Infection in pregnancy may result in fetal loss or congenital rubella syndrome (cataracts and other eye defects, deafness, cardiac abnormalities, microcephaly, inflammatory lesions of brain, liver, lungs and bone marrow). Infection in the first 8–10 weeks of pregnancy results in damage to up to 90% of surviving infants, with multiple defects being common. The risk of damage in the later stages of pregnancy declines and except for deafness, fetal damage is rare after 16 weeks.

In the UK and elsewhere, prepubertal girls and non-immune women of child-bearing age were routinely immunized to prevent rubella infection in pregnancy. Selective vaccination of teenage girls ceased in 1996. This has been replaced with the MMR vaccine, which is administered to infants and adults of both sexes with the long-term aim of eradicating these diseases from the population. Rubella infection levels in the UK are currently so low they are defined as eliminated by the World Health Organization. Therefore, routine screening of pregnant women for rubella susceptibility ceased in 2016 in the UK. MMR is given in over 100 countries, including those in the European Union. In Finland, a two-dose MMR schedule was introduced in 1982. As a result of persistently high vaccine coverage of the population, indigenous MMR was eliminated from Finland in 1994 and has not returned. Rubella has been eliminated from Cuba and the USA.

The guidance on administrating live vaccines together has recently been revised and is now based on the specific vaccine combinations. The rationale for avoiding simultaneous vaccination with two live vaccines relates to the production of natural interferon in response to a live vaccine. If a second live vaccine is given during this response period, the interferon may prevent replication of the second vaccine virus and the subsequent antibody response and vaccine efficacy may be diminished. For example, if there is no pressing reason to give the vaccines on the same day, varicella vaccine and MMR are administered at least four weeks apart. If a tuberculin skin test has already been initiated, then MMR should be delayed until the skin test has been read unless protection against measles is required urgently.

Varicella immunization

Chickenpox (varicella) is caused by the varicella zoster virus and is highly infectious. The infection can occur at any age but is more common in children. However, disease in adults tends to be more severe. The primary infection presents initially with itchy blisters on the skin that later scab and may cause scarring. The virus eventually becomes latent in the sensory ganglion (nerve cells) but can reactivate later in life as shingles (herpes zoster), resulting in a painful, vesicular (blistering) skin rash. Whether in the primary or the reactivation secondary form of the disease, vesicles contain virus and are infectious.

If a woman is infected with chickenpox whilst pregnant, there are risks to both her and the baby. Chickenpox can cause severe maternal disease, and 10–20% of pregnant women infected later in pregnancy may develop varicella pneumonia, which can be fatal. During the first 20 weeks of pregnancy, chickenpox infection in the mother can occasionally cause damage to the fetus (congenital varicella syndrome), stillbirth or shingles during infancy. Fortunately, this is an uncommon occurrence affecting about 1–2% of fetuses. A newborn baby may also be infected if the mother develops chickenpox during the perinatal period. Newborn babies whose mothers develop a varicella rash between five days before to two days after delivery are at risk of neonatal varicella, and approximately 30% of these babies may die. The high mortality is thought to be due to the newborn baby not receiving transplacental antibodies from the mother coupled with the immaturity of the baby's immune system.

Recommendations for varicella vaccination

Approximately 10% of the population have no immunity to varicella (chickenpox). Varicella is transmitted directly by personal contact or droplet spread, and in household contacts the secondary infection rate from a case of chickenpox can be as high as 90%. Vaccination protects both susceptible healthcare workers and vulnerable patients, such as pregnant women or the immunosuppressed, who might acquire chickenpox from an infected member of staff. Staff or students who have no previous history of chickenpox or shingles should have a blood test to check their immunity; if seronegative, then vaccination is recommended. If there is a definite history of chickenpox or shingles, the person can be considered to be immune. A recent survey showed that a history of chickenpox is a less reliable predictor of immunity in individuals born and raised overseas and routine testing should be considered. Immunization comprises two doses of the live attenuated vaccine 4–8 weeks apart. Varicella vaccine is contraindicated in pregnancy and as a precaution, pregnancy should be avoided for one month following the last dose of varicella vaccine. An American surveillance registry started in 1995 that monitors pregnancy outcomes following inadvertent vaccination of pregnant women has not identified any vaccine-associated risk to the fetus. Please note the occupational varicella vaccine differs from the herpes zoster vaccine used for the prevention of shingles in the elderly, which is formulated at a higher dose to compensate for the waning of the immune system with age.

Syphilis

Since the beginning of this century, syphilis has re-emerged due to outbreaks originating in major cities across Europe. The majority of cases are in men who have sex with men, though smaller numbers of heterosexual women, including pregnant women, have also been infected. Syphilis can cross the placenta and infect the fetus. Anonymous antenatal serological testing in England in 2014 showed that 0.14% of pregnant women screened positive for syphilis.

Oral sex was identified as the route of transmission in approximately 40% of the notified cases. Dentists should refer any patients with suspicious lesions suggestive of either primary syphilis (presenting as a chancre – an indurated ulcer) or secondary syphilis (presenting as oral ulceration and/or mucosal lesions) to the patient's medical practitioner or their local sexual health clinic. Syphilis is most infectious during the primary and secondary stages of the disease. In terms of occupational exposures, a dental healthcare worker could acquire a syphilis infection if an abrasion or cut on their skin came into contact with a syphilitic lesion in a patient with primary or secondary syphilis present on the lips or oral mucosa. Fortunately, like condoms, surgical gloves provide an effective barrier to transmission. Although blood-borne transmission via needlestick injury has been documented, the amount of *Treponema pallidum* in blood is very small, and transmission of syphilis from even high-risk sharps injuries is extremely rare. Antibiotic prophylaxis is available following occupational exposure and prompt advice should be sought from the local occupational health department.

OCCUPATIONAL VACCINES TO PROTECT AGAINST HEPATITIS AND TB

Since the introduction of routine hepatitis B vaccine for healthcare workers and students, the number of cases of occupationally acquired hepatitis B has fallen dramatically. Since 2004, in the UK there have been no cases of occupational transmission of HBV cases due to sharps or splash incidents.

There are two classes of products available for occupational immunization against hepatitis B: a vaccine that confers active immunity and hepatitis B immunoglobulin (HBIG) that provides passive and temporary immunity for those at high risk of infection following a sharps injury. Postexposure prophylaxis against hepatitis B is discussed in Chapter 4.

Hepatitis B vaccine

Hepatitis B vaccine contains hepatitis B surface antigen (HBsAg), and is prepared from yeast cells using recombinant DNA technology. As the vaccine contains inactivated virus, it is very safe and is incapable of causing hepatitis.

A standard vaccine course consists of three immunizations that stimulate the production of specific antibodies to HBsAg. Approximately 10–15% of adults fail to respond to three doses of vaccine or respond poorly. Vaccine failures or poor responses are mostly associated with age over 40 years, obesity, smoking and immunosuppression. HBV vaccine is ineffective in patients with acute hepatitis B, and is not necessary for individuals known to have markers of current infection (HBsAg) or antibodies showing evidence of past hepatitis B infection.

Antibody response to the vaccine is measured 1–4 months after completing the course of immunization to ensure that an adequate antibody (hepatitis B surface antibody titre (HBsAb) ≥100 IU/mL) response has been mounted and the titre recorded. Antibody responses vary widely between individuals. In the UK, HBsAb levels at or above 10 IU/mL are generally accepted as offering protect against infection; HBsAb levels greater than 100 IU/mL are consistent with a good immune response.

Maximum antibody titres are usually found one month after completing the course with a rapid decline over the next 12 months and thereafter the titre falls more slowly. Immunological memory ensures that protection against infection is sustained even though the circulating concentration of antibodies declines with time. However, recent evidence suggests that not all individuals may respond in this way and the full duration of protection afforded by hepatitis B vaccine has yet to be completely established. Therefore, dental personnel at continuing risk of infection should be offered a single booster (reinforcing) dose of vaccine around five years after the primary course of immunization. A further assessment of antibody levels is not indicated. If a reinforcing dose is given before five years for postexposure prophylaxis then a second reinforcing dose at five years is not required.

Poor responders and non-responders

Poor responders with an antibody response of between 10 and 100 IU/mL should be offered an additional dose of vaccine as this may improve the initial antibody titre. They should also receive the standard reinforcing dose at five years as recommended above.

Non-responders to hepatitis B vaccine

A healthcare worker with an antibody titre below 10 IU/mL is classified as a non-responder to the vaccine, and such people are then tested for markers of current or past infection with HBV. Vaccine non-responders may have natural immunity to hepatitis B due to past infection from which they have fully recovered and cleared the virus. Alternatively, they may be asymptomatic carriers of hepatitis B. Both groups do not respond to the vaccine and for employment health clearance, it is essential to determine which category the dental healthcare worker or student falls into. True non-responders are normally offered a repeat course of immunization. This is followed by retesting 1–4 months after the second course. If they fail to mount an adequate antibody response, and remain non-responders, they can continue to perform exposure-prone procedures (EPPs). However, should a non-responder have a sharps injury or splash incident and there is a risk of exposure to HBV, they will require prompt referral to the local accident and emergency department/occupational health department for hepatitis B immunoglobulin.

BCG vaccine

Tuberculosis is caused by infection with *Mycobacterium tuberculosis*. The most common form is pulmonary TB, which accounts for approximately 50% of all cases in the UK, although *M. tuberculosis* can affect almost every part of the body. General symptoms include fever, unexplained fatigue, significant weight loss, night sweats and a persistent cough for more than three weeks, accompanied by blood-stained sputum and enlarged lymph nodes (particularly cervical nodes). In Europe, most cases are acquired through the respiratory route. TB is not an inevitable result of infection with the bacterium. The spectrum of tuberculosis infection shows a dynamic multistate gradient that includes:

- an ability to mount effective immune responses that eradicate all viable TB bacilli
- an immune response able to contain the infection but the individual continues to harbour populations of bacilli that intermittently replicate in macrophages, granulomata and other tissues (latent subclinical infection)
- lack of effective immunity against TB and rapid progress from tuberculosis infection to disease, e.g. young children, the chronically ill, immunosuppressed and HIV-infected people.

Virtually all episodes of tuberculosis disease are preceded by a period of asymptomatic infection which can persist for years. The majority of TB cases in the UK are the result of 'reactivation' of latent TB infection (LTBI) so that the onset of TB can be insidious and difficult to detect with significant diagnostic delays. Late diagnoses are associated with worse outcomes for the individual and, in the case of pulmonary TB, with a transmission risk to the public. Therefore, identifying and treating people with latent subclinical infections in order to prevent future disease provides a crucial opportunity to interrupt TB transmission and thereby reduce the national and global burden of tuberculosis disease (see Chapter 2).

Latent TB infection can be diagnosed by a single blood test (interferon-gamma release assay – IGRA), and is usually treated with antibiotics. LTBI testing and treatment is recommend for 16–35 year olds who recently arrived in England from high-incidence countries where TB incidence is ≥150/100 000 population or sub-Saharan Africa. Several conditions may co-exist with LTBI and may increase a person's likelihood of TB, including HIV infection, alcoholic liver disease, malnutrition, diabetes mellitus, renal dialysis and immunosuppressive therapies. In the case of healthcare workers with LTBI, there are no age restrictions for prescribing chemoprophylaxis treatment, either six months of isoniazid or three months of isoniazid/rifampicin combination therapy.

Up until 2005 in the UK, schoolchildren were vaccinated against TB at the age of 12–14 years. This programme has now been replaced with a targeted, risk-based immunization protocol for susceptible neonates. Consequently, most dental trainees will not have received the BCG vaccination prior to entering training.

Studies examining the effectiveness of BCG vaccine from across the world have reported wide variations, from no protection to 60–80% protection in UK schoolchildren. Recent data suggest that BCG vaccination protects against *M. tuberculosis* infection as well as progression from infection to disease in children. BCG efficacy against pulmonary disease shows geographic variation, and pulmonary disease is more common in adults. The vaccine does not seem to protect those people already infected or sensitized to environmental mycobacteria. Vaccine protection may wane over time, but is normally considered effective for about 10–15 years.

Healthcare workers are more likely than the general population to come into contact with someone with TB. BCG vaccination is recommended for all clinical dental healthcare personnel and students who have close contact with patients, are Mantoux tuberculin skin test (or interferon-gamma test) negative and have not been previously vaccinated.

HEALTH CHECKS AND THE CONSEQUENCES OF BLOOD-BORNE VIRUS INFECTION

A healthcare worker is defined as an individual who has direct clinical contact with a patient. All dental healthcare workers and dental, therapist and hygienist students entering the health service for the first time, and dental healthcare workers rejoining after a period of absence are obliged to complete statutory standard precourse enrolment or pre-employment health clearance checks. Each person is individually risk assessed based on the clinical procedures outlined in their job description or training curriculum by an occupational health service. Those undertaking EPPs will require additional health screening tests. The purpose of these recommendations is not to restrict healthcare workers infected with blood-borne virus (BBV) from working but to restrict them from undertaking EPPs where their infection status may pose a risk to patients in their care.

Exposure-prone procedures – 'bleed-back'

An exposure-prone procedure or unrecognized bleed-back into the patient's open tissues is defined by UKAP as follows:

> EPPs include procedures where the worker's gloved hands may be in contact with sharp instruments, needle tips or sharp tissues inside a patient's open body cavity, wound or confined anatomical space where the hands or fingertips may not be completely visible at all times.

The term exposure-prone procedure embraces a wide range of general dental and surgical procedures, in which there may be very different levels of bleedback risk. They are classified into three risk-based categories depending on the degree of visibility of the hands and the risk of significant percutaneous injury occurring during the procedure. General dental treatment performed in primary care may be categorized as either non-EPP and have a negligible risk of bleedback or fall within EPP categories 1 and 2 with increasing risk of bleed-back. Certain maxillofacial surgical procedures are defined as category 3 (see Table 3.2 for examples in each of the categories). In addition, UKAP guidelines state that 'Other situations, such as pre-hospital trauma care, should be avoided by HCWs restricted from performing EPPs, as they could also result in the exposure of the patient's open tissues to the blood of the worker'.

HEALTH CLEARANCE

Standard health clearance

It is current policy in the NHS and private dental care to screen healthcare workers on appointment for:

- TB immunity (evidence of tuberculin skin test or interferon-gamma testing and/or BCG scar checked by an occupational health professional)
- offer of hepatitis B immunization, with postimmunization testing of response
- offer of testing for hepatitis C and HIV, in the context of reminding healthcare workers of their professional responsibilities in relation to serious communicable disease.

Employees or students new to dentistry who will be working with patients should not start work until they have completed a TB screen or health check, or until documentary evidence is provided of such screening having taken place within the preceding 12 months. The risk of TB for a new healthcare worker who knows he or she is HIV positive at the time of recruitment should be assessed as part of the occupational health checks, as they may need to modify their clinical work to reduce the risk of TB exposure. Dental healthcare personnel

Table 3.2 Classification of exposure-prone procedures (EPPs) and non-EPPs

Category	Definition	Associated risk	Examples of procedures
1	Procedures where the hands and fingertips of the worker are usually visible and outside the body most of the time and the possibility of injury to the worker's gloved hands from sharp instruments and/or tissues is slight	Low	Local anaesthetic injections Polishing of teeth or restorations using finishing burs in high-speed handpieces
2	Procedures where the fingertips may not be visible at all times but injury to the worker's gloved hands from sharp instruments and/or tissues is unlikely	Intermediate	Extraction of a tooth Root canal therapy
3	Procedures where the fingertips are out of sight for a significant part of the procedure, or during certain critical stages, and in which there is a distinct risk of injury to the worker's gloved hands from sharp instruments and/or tissues	Highest	Osteotomy
Non-EPP	Procedures where the hands and fingertips of the worker are visible and outside the patient's body at all times, and internal examinations or procedures do not involve possible injury to the worker's gloved hands from sharp instruments and/or tissues	Are considered not to be exposure prone provided routine infection prevention and control procedures are adhered to at all times	Incision of external abscesses Taking impressions

Based on PHE. General Dentistry Exposure Prone Procedure (EPP) Categorization. Advice from the United Kingdom Advisory Panel for Healthcare Workers Infected with Bloodborne Viruses (UKAP). A full list of examples of EPPs and non-EPPs is available from UKAP.

and students for whom hepatitis B vaccination is contraindicated, who decline vaccination or who are non-responders to vaccine should be restricted from performing EPPs unless shown to be non-infectious (i.e. negative for hepatitis B surface antigen). Periodic retesting may need to be considered.

Additional health checks

All dental healthcare workers who perform EPPs (such as dentists, therapists and hygienists) must have pre-employment additional health checks that are to be completed prior to confirmation of their post. All potential undergraduate dental students and dental therapist and hygienist students must undergo additional health clearance before acceptance onto the course. They will be ineligible to perform EPPs if found to be infectious until successfully treated and appropriately monitored. International students transferring to the UK will need to conform to the same testing arrangements as new entrants to dental school, prior to undertaking EPPs.

Students who are identified as HBV or HIV positive but who achieve clearance for EPPs on the basis of viral suppression with antiviral agents must be made aware of the long-term career implications should viral breakthrough occur. Tests performed abroad must be repeated in the UK and only the UK result will be accepted. Laboratory test results required for clearance to perform EPPs must be derived from an identified validated sample (IVS), i.e. one obtained in occupational health and sent directly to the laboratory (to avoid an individual exchanging their blood for that of another individual known to be of low risk).

The dental healthcare workers or students/trainees performing EPPs must be:

- hepatitis B surface antigen negative or, if positive, e-antigen negative with a viral load of less than $200\,IU/mL$ (either from natural suppression or 12 months after cessation of antiviral therapy) or have a viral load of less than $200\,IU/mL$ whilst on continuous antiviral therapy (if their pretreatment viral load was 200–$20\,000\,IU/mL$)
- hepatitis C antibody negative (or HCV RNA negative either as a consequence of natural clearance or six months after cessation of antiviral therapy)
- non-infectious for HIV (either antibody negative or on effective combination antiretroviral therapy and having a plasma viral load <200 copies/mL, or be an elite controller).

These viral titres reflect both threshold levels of virus needed to initiate infection and innovations in antiviral treatment. In order to be permitted to perform EPPs, staff and students who are HBsAg positive and HBeAg negative must also comply with the following measures.

- Be subject to plasma viral load monitoring every three months whilst on continuous viral therapy; or annually if they have a viral load of $<200\,IU/mL$ either from natural suppression or 12 months after cessation of antiviral therapy.
- Be under joint supervision of their treating physician and a consultant occupational health physician.
- Be registered with the UKAP Occupational Health Monitoring Register of Blood-Borne Infected HCWs (UKAP-OHR).

Students returning from overseas elective period projects in areas where BBVs are common may require retesting through an occupational health department if they may have been inadvertently exposed in a high-risk setting. Dental students who are successfully treated for BBV infection and who are appropriately monitored for HIV and HBV will normally become eligible to perform EPPs.

HIV-infected healthcare workers

Since HIV was first diagnosed in 1981, in the developed world there has only been one documented case of an HIV-positive dentist who was alleged to have infected his patients. The case in question is the much-publicized 1990 Dr Acer case in Florida, USA. The dentist infected six of his patients. Even after extensive investigations costing $4 million, the method by which HIV was transmitted was never discovered. In the UK and elsewhere, there have been a number of look-back patient notification exercises involving patients who had received treatment from dentists who were subsequently found to be HIV positive. None of these exercises has ever shown HIV transmission from the clinician to the patient as a result of dental treatment.

During the intervening years, protocols for infection control have been significantly upgraded and enforced, thereby increasing protection of the public. The infectivity of patients living with HIV and therefore the associated risk involved in treating such patients has dramatically decreased with the introduction of effective combination antiretroviral treatment (cART), which can produce an undetectable viral load. In 1991, the US Centers for Disease Control and Prevention announced that mandatory testing and restriction of work procedures were not recommended for HIV-positive healthcare workers, provided they adhered to standard precautions for infection control and used safety equipment and needles (see Chapter 5). This relaxation of the regulations did not result in any new cases. Since 2014 in the UK, HIV-positive healthcare workers are permitted to treat patients undergoing EPPs as long as they comply with the following guidance.

- On effective cART and have a plasma viral load <200 copies/mL (or be an elite controller with a viral load of <200 copies/mL).
- Be subject to plasma viral load monitoring every three months.
- Be under joint supervision of their treating physician and a consultant occupational health physician.
- Be registered with the UKAP-OHR.

DUTY OF CARE TO PATIENTS

Dentists or other dental healthcare personnel currently registered with the GDC who believe that they may have been exposed to blood-borne viruses are under a legal, professional and ethical obligation to promptly seek and follow confidential advice on testing for BBV and national guidelines on practising restrictions. Failure to do so may breach the duty of care to patients under the Health and Safety at Work Act and the Control of Substances Hazardous to Health Regulations and the conditions of registration with the GDC. Such a breach might constitute 'a fitness to practise' concern, depending on the specific circumstances.

Antidiscrimination legislation

Over the years, as new infections emerged, fear over the consequences of becoming infected with a BBV made some members of the dental profession reluctant to treat infected patients in primary dental care, and to refer patients to the hospital sector for treatment. Patients who have contracted HIV, HBV or HCV or any other blood-borne viruses are entitled to receive dental treatment. However, in exceptional circumstances government bodies will introduce preventive measures to curb the spread of disease. For example, during the Ebola outbreak in 2013–15, restrictions were placed on returning healthcare workers who had volunteered to treat Ebola patients in West Africa from receiving elective routine dentistry in primary dental care during the incubation period of the disease.

Patients' rights are protected in the GDC's *Standards for Dental Professional*: 'Standard 1.6 You must treat patients fairly, as individuals and without discrimination, which includes not discriminating against patients on the grounds of race, sexual orientation, sex, disability or health'. In Britain, the Equality Act 2010 provides the legal framework to protect patients from discrimination or unfair treatment by healthcare providers based on one of the protected characteristics under the Act: age, disability, gender reassignment, pregnancy or maternity, race, religion or belief, sex and sexual orientation.

REFERENCES AND WEBSITES

Bailey E, Tickle M, Campbell S. (2014) Patient safety in primary care dentistry: where are we now? *British Dental Journal*, **217**, 339–344.

Public Health England (2013) Immunization Against Infectious Disease – 'The Green Book', 3rd edn. Available at: www.gov.uk/government/collections/immunization-against-infectious-disease-the-green-book (accessed 27 October 2016).

Public Health England (2014) The Management of HIV Infected Healthcare Workers Who Perform Exposure Prone Procedures: Updated Guidance. Available at: www.gov.uk/government/uploads/system/uploads/attachment_data/file/333018/Management_of_HIV_infected_Healthcare_Workers_guidance_January_2014.pdf (accessed 27 October 2016).

Public Health England (2016) General Dentistry Exposure Prone Procedure (EPP) Categorization. Advice from the United Kingdom Advisory Panel for Healthcare Workers Infected with Bloodborne Viruses (UKAP). Available at: www.gov.uk/

government/publications/general-dentistry-exposure-prone-procedure-categorisation (accessed 27 October 2016).

Rangaka MX, Cavalcante SC, Marais BJ *et al.* (2015) Controlling the seedbeds of tuberculosis: diagnosis and treatment of tuberculosis infection. *Lancet,* **386,** 2344–2453.

Woode OM, Wellington E, Rice B *et al.* (2014) Eye of the Needle. United Kingdom Surveillance of Significant Occupational Exposures to Bloodborne Viruses in Healthcare Workers. Available at: www.gov.uk/government/publications/blood borne-viruses-eye-of-the-needle (accessed 27 October 2016).

Chapter 4

Sharp safe working in the dental surgery

WHY SHARPS PREVENTION IS IMPORTANT

Sharps injuries and splashes to eyes or broken skin can transmit BBV infections.

A sharps injury refers to any injury or puncture to the skin involving a sharp instrument, such as a dental bur, syringe needle or suture needle. Percutaneous injuries (including human bites) often produce only a minor injury to the skin, but they are clinically significant as they can transmit blood-borne viruses (BBVs), namely hepatitis C (HCV), hepatitis B (HBV) and human immunodeficiency virus (HIV). BBVs can enter the tissues and cause infection following splashes into the eye, oral mucosa or on to broken skin (abrasions, cuts, eczema, etc.); however, the risk of transmission by these routes is considerably lower than for sharps injuries. Intact skin forms a barrier to BBV transmission and infection does not occur through inhalation or via the faecal–oral route.

In the dental surgery, the most common route for transmission of a BBV infection is from an infected patient to a clinician. An infectious dental patient may not necessarily be identified from their medical history if they are an asymptomatic carrier. Such people are often blissfully unaware of their condition.

Infrequently, a BBV-infected healthcare worker will infect a patient, or very rarely transmission occurs from patient to patient via contaminated instruments or environmental surfaces. Look-back investigations of HBV outbreaks revealed that transmission tended to occur when the source person was highly contagious due to a high viral load in their bloodstream, coupled with a breakdown in standard infection control precautions. A dramatic illustration of this

Basic Guide to Infection Prevention and Control in Dentistry, Second Edition.
Caroline L. Pankhurst.
© 2017 John Wiley & Sons Ltd. Published 2017 by John Wiley & Sons Ltd.
Companion website: www.wiley.com/go/pankhurst/infection-prevention

type of scenario is an outbreak of hepatitis B centred on an HBe antigen-positive dentist with acute hepatitis B who continued working. He infected 6.9% of the patients attending his practice. Patients were infected only at the times when he omitted to wear gloves during dental treatment (Hadler *et al.*, 1981). Fortunately, occupational acquisition of HBV by healthcare workers (HCWs) has declined dramatically over the past three decades because of the introduction of hepatitis B vaccination and increased adherence to standard infection control precautions (SICPs).

Across most of Western Europe, the prevalence of BBV in the general population is comparatively low but the numbers are increasing year on year. In the USA, 3.2 million people have chronic HCV and 1.2 million chronic HBV. In the UK, an estimated 214 000 people are living with chronic HCV and just over 100 000 people are living with HIV. The practical implication of these statistics is that most dental practices will have a small number of BBV seropositive patients.

Following a single percutaneous injury, especially a deep penetrating injury with a scalpel, a hollow-bore needle, aspirating syringe or a device visibly contaminated with blood, the probability of seroconverting is estimated at:

- 1 in 3 for HBV
- 1 in 30 for HCV
- 1 in 300 for HIV
- 1 in 1000 for HIV for mucocutaneous (mucous membranes and skin) splashing.

An alternative way of looking at these figures is that hepatitis B is 100 times and hepatitis C is 10 times more likely to be transmitted than HIV in the dental setting. The actual risk of seroconversion is dependent on:

- prevalence of the infection in the local population
- how infectious the patient is (i.e. stage of illness or current antiviral treatment)
- whether the dental treatment or task is likely to result in a sharps injury or splash.

Overall, because of the low prevalence rates of BBV infections in the UK, the risk to dental staff or students of acquiring a BBV occupationally is small.

Since 1997 an ongoing national surveillance study called 'Eye of the Needle' has been conducted in the UK to measure actual rates of HBV, HCV and HIV seroconversion in healthcare staff following occupational sharps injuries. In healthcare workers reporting a significant occupational exposure, half were exposed to HCV, a third to HIV and one in 10 to HBV. During the first eight years of the survey, there were five cases (0.48%) of occupationally acquired HIV infection, and 11 (1.8%) healthcare personnel seroconverted to HCV, one of whom was a dentist. In contrast, from 2004 to 2013 due to improvements in sharp safe working, HBV immunization and management of sharps injuries, no healthcare workers in the UK acquired HIV or HBV occupationally and only nine HCWs seroconverted to HCV. Worryingly, nearly 50% of the incidents that involved members of the dental team were preventable; 39% of exposures occurred after the dental procedure but before disposal. Preventable injuries were higher in dentistry than in any other sector of healthcare. Most of the preventable injuries in dentistry affect dental care partners, occurring whilst clearing the bracket table, disposing of needles and during manual cleaning of instruments. Incidents are more likely to involve sharp hand instruments rather than needles. Later in the chapter we will look at the new regulations introduced in the UK and across the member states of the European Union to reduce sharps injuries in all healthcare personnel and students, and describe other practical solutions to reducing preventable injuries.

Although the BBV seroconversion rates are low, nobody in dentistry can afford to be complacent about the way they work, because of the serious and sometimes life-threatening consequences of a BBV infection. These have an impact not only on their own health and ability to work but also on the practitioner's partners as the BBV can be transmitted sexually and to the unborn child (see Chapter 2 for routes of transmission of BBV). Cross-infection risks for patients arising from HCV or HBV seropositive staff who knowingly breach regulations on clinical practice can jeopardize the reputation of the dental practice, and have significant financial knock-on effects on colleagues (see Chapter 3). As a matter of routine, you must regard all blood and blood-tainted body fluids, e.g. saliva, as potentially infectious, and apply SICPs.

WHEN DO SHARPS INJURIES OCCUR?

Half of sharps injuries are preventable.

Surveys evaluating sharps injuries affecting American and Scottish dental practitioners found that on average, they sustained 1.7–3.5 sharps injuries per year. We know that as many as a third of dentists are reluctant to report sharps injuries, so these figures may be an underestimate. In the Scottish study, 30% of the dentists' injuries constituted a significant exposure (i.e. source patient, HIV, HBV, HCV seropositive). A small proportion of documented injuries involve the use of increased force, bending needles or passing of sharp instruments between the dentist and the nurse, whereas most intraoral needlestick and sharps injuries occur accidentally during the course of routine treatment as a result of sudden unexpected patient movements, closing the mouth, or as a consequence of poor visibility. Such incidents are intrinsic to working in the confines of the mouth. While they can be reduced to a degree by training, behavioural changes and engineering innovations, they cannot be completely eliminated.

SHARP SAFE WORKING IN THE DENTAL SURGERY

PREVENTABLE SHARPS INJURIES

Never leave unsheathed needles on the bracket table.

Most needlestick injuries happen outside the mouth, during resheathing, dismantling or disposal of needles. Such needlestick injuries are considered 'avoidable' with safe practice. Preventive measures such as the use of safety sharps that incorporate an integral safety mechanism within the design, such as a retractable sheath, were demonstrated to significantly reduce extraoral injuries. 'Sharp-less surgical techniques' that use electric scalpels, glues and clips are advocated as a safer alternative to sutures and scalpels.

Clearing up dental instruments at the end of treatment and manual cleaning are fraught with opportunities for sharps injuries unless precautions are taken. It is during these activities that dental nurses are most at risk. Injuries are usually sustained by the non-dominant hand. Forty percent of extraoral injuries involve dental burs and probe tips. Fortunately, these instruments are usually less heavily contaminated with blood than hollow-bore needles and so pose less of a risk for transmission of infection. Even if they do not result in an infection, sharps injuries can lead to considerable distress for the victim, resulting in sickness absence, and may require counseling to restore loss of confidence and self-esteem.

Employers are required to protect their staff from exposure to sharps injuries and BBV exposure under the Health and Safety (Sharp Instruments in Healthcare) Regulations 2013 (Box 4.1) which builds upon existing legislation in Britain and Northern Ireland, including the Health and Social Care Act Approved Code of Practice and Control of Substances Hazardous to Health Regulations (see Chapter 1).

HOW TO AVOID A SHARPS INJURY

Safe disposal of needles and scalpels is the responsibility of the clinician.

Safe handling of sharps

Injuries associated with handling and disposal of sharps and clinical sharps waste can be minimized by adhering to accepted good practice.

Good practice guide: sharp safe dental treatment
- Use an instrument (mirror/cheek retractor) rather than fingers to retract tongue and cheeks when using sharp implements. This has the added advantage of enhancing visibility.

> ## Box 4.1 Summary of key duties and obligation for employers and employees from the Health and Safety (Sharp Instruments in Healthcare) Regulations 2013
>
> **Regulations place specific obligations on healthcare employers and contractors to protect employees from injuries caused by medical sharps by:**
> - conducting risk assessments
> - avoiding unnecessary use of sharps and where this is not possible, using safer sharps that incorporate a protection mechanism
> - preventing the recapping of needles (dentistry is exempt based on risk assessments, but employer must provide safety device if recapping, e.g. safety sharps)
> - ensuring safe disposal by placing secure sharps containers close to the point of use
> - providing employees with adequate information and training on the safe use and disposal of sharps
> - providing employees with training and instructions on what to do in the event of a sharps injury and on the local arrangements for postexposure testing, immunization and postexposure prophylaxis, if required
> - recording and investigating sharps incidents
> - providing employees who have been injured with access to medical advice, and offering testing, immunization, postexposure prophylaxis and counseling, when required.
>
> **Obligations of employees:**
> - employees who receive a sharps injury whilst undertaking their work must inform their employer as soon as is practicable
> - healthcare workers must be aware of their responsibility in avoiding sharps injuries.
>
> *Source*: Based on European Council Directive 2010/32/EU.

- Do not bend the local anaesthetic needle (as this interferes with resheathing and is more likely to lead to injury) (Figure 4.1).
- Avoid recapping needles where possible and only recap using a safety needle with a retractable sheath or other incorporated safety device. If these are unavailable, use a needle block or needle guard (Figure 4.2).
- Never resheath needles using an unprotected hand.
- Avoid passing sharp instruments from hand to hand during dental treatment. The same sharp instrument should not be touched by more than one person at the same time. Place the sharp in a neutral zone in the tray or bracket table from where it can safely be picked up by the second person. Alert the other person that you are putting a sharp instrument into the neutral zone.

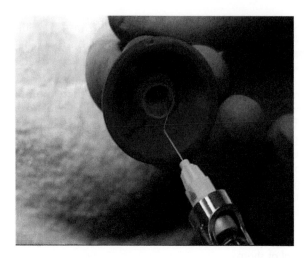

Figure 4.1 Illustration to show the difficulty in removing a bent needle with a needle guard.

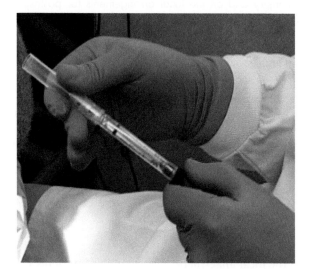

Figure 4.2 Safety needle with integral retractable sheath, shown in safe position; sheath is withdrawn for giving the local anaesthetic.

Use of safety sharps

Dentistry is unique in its continuing deployment of reusable metal syringes rather than plastic disposable syringes. They are potentially dangerous devices as resheathing and needle disassembly are undertaken at a time when the needle is contaminated with blood. Recent innovations in the design of syringes and other sharps aim to minimize both clinical and 'downstream' injuries associated with cleaning and disposing of sharps that affect nurses and cleaners.

Safety needles with integrated retractable sheath – the sheath can be retracted whenever the needle is required to give an injection and is then slid down over the needle, protecting the operator between use and during dismantling and disposal (see Figure 4.2). Some syringe and needle devices are fully disposable as a single unit, which minimizes the degree of handling

Free-standing needle guards and resheathing blocks are designed to protect the hand that is used to recap the needle but are not as effective as an incorporated safety device (see Figure 4.2). Since 2013, according to changes in UK and European law, these devices are no longer the method of choice where a safety sharp is available, but may still be deployed as the norm elsewhere.

A review of needlestick injuries across the health service in Scotland suggested that 56% of injuries would 'probably' or 'definitely' have been prevented if a safety device had been used (Young *et al.*, 2007). At a dental school in London, following an introductory training course in the use of the safety syringes, the number of avoidable needlestick injuries sustained by dental students fell from 11.8 injuries/million hours worked/year down to zero (Zakrzewska *et al.*, 2001).

Sharp safe disposal

Good practice guide: safe disposal of sharps and needles
- Single-use sharps should be discarded immediately after use by the user.
- *Never* leave sharps on the bracket table to be disposed of by someone else as this is when accidents occur.
- Use disposable safety scalpels, which avoid the need to release the blade (Figure 4.3).
- Do not leave burs in the handpiece at the end of treatment as they can catch on skin and clothing. The clinician should remove them immediately after use and then the handpiece can be dismantled from the connector and cleaned without the risk of injury to the nurse.
- Place disposable sharps directly into a rigid puncture-proof yellow-lidded waste receptacle (bin).
- When using a disposable syringe and needle, discard as one unit directly into a sharps bin.

Good practice guide: assembly and use of sharps receptacles
- Ensure that the sharps bin is correctly assembled and that the lid is securely fastened before commencing use.
- Place bins conveniently close to the point of use. Wall mount or insert into sturdy non-tip base plate.
- Do not place sharps bins on the floor, on an unstable surface or above shoulder height.

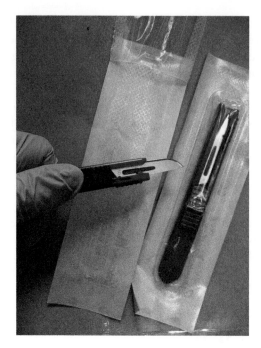

Figure 4.3 Disposable retractable scalpel blade shown in the open position for use and in the safety position within the integral sheath.

- Keep the aperture closed when the sharps bin is not in use (Figure 4.4).
- Seal and dispose of when three-quarters full (do not attempt to press down on contents to make more room!).
- Never try to retrieve any items from a sharps bin.

MANAGING SHARPS INJURIES AND SPLASHES

It is a requirement under the Health and Social Care Act Approved Code of Practice 2015 that all healthcare workers should have access to immediate, 24-hour management of sharps injuries. Occupational injury assessment is provided either by the local occupational health department or, if this service is unavailable, by the nearest accident and emergency department. In order to avoid unnecessary delays, the telephone number and name of the appropriate contact person should be made known to all the staff working at the practice. Under the COSHH regulations, employers must ensure that all their staff are aware of the action to be taken following a sharps or splash incident. This includes immediate first aid, reporting procedures and further management (Figure 4.5). The procedure will vary depending on whether or not the source patient can be identified. An example of a sharps incident occurring on an unknown source are those injuries that occur during manual cleaning of pooled

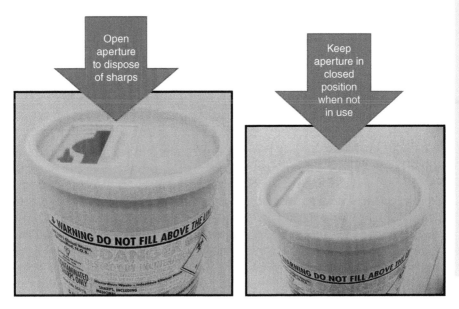

Figure 4.4 Aperture of the sharps receptacle shown in the open and closed positions.

Percutaneous sharps injury: encourage puncture site to bleed by applying pressure (<u>do not suck</u>).
- Wash site liberally with soap and running water for several minutes
- Do not scrub as this may inoculate virus into the tissues
- Cover with a waterproof plaster

Splash to eyes: thoroughly wash eye with running water or eye washsolution (remove contact lens prior to washing eyes)

Splash exposure of oral mucous membranes: Rinse vigorously withwater and spit out

- Report incident *immediately*
- Recheck patient's medical history and ask about risk behaviours for BBV
- Arrange for blood sample to be taken from donor for testing

- Promptly contact (local Occupational Health Department / Accident & Emergency Department) for urgent risk assessment of injury, information and counselling
- Administer post exposure prophylaxis according to risk assessment

- Complete an Accident Report form

Figure 4.5 Immediate first aid and further management following a percutaneous or splash incident.

instruments from several patients. In either case the injured healthcare worker should stop work at once and report the incident immediately.

OCCUPATIONAL HEALTH RISK ASSESSMENT FOR BBV EXPOSURE

If the source patient is known, then inform the source patient and ask them to wait in surgery, in order that the patient's medical history and risk behaviours for BBV can be reviewed, and the person in charge can make arrangements with the donor's general medical practitioner for a blood sample to be taken and tested. To ensure the patient's co-operation, it is important that the infection control lead/ registered provider/manager (preferably not the exposed person) should explain about the incident and why the additional enquiries and blood tests are being sought. The patient should be reassured that strict confidentiality will be maintained throughout the process. The source patient should receive a pretest discussion (occupational and personal implications of a positive test) and give informed consent for a blood sample to be taken for HIV, HBV and HCV testing. In some instances, additional serological testing may be required, for example for HTLV-1.

However, outside a dental hospital setting it may be difficult to arrange for a blood sample to be taken on the same day. In such cases, the staff member should not delay in contacting the occupational health service for advice. The risk assessment is then based on the available information, including patient's history, type of injury, presence of blood on the instrument and the background rate of infection in the local community. The patient's responses to the questions outlined in Box 4.2 should be recorded in the accident logbook.

How the incident is assessed and subsequently managed will be modified according to the immune status of the recipient, and if the exposure was significant (with the potential to transmit BBV). Individual responses will inform the decision on whether or not to administer HIV prophylaxis and/or a booster immunization of hepatitis B or immunoglobulin (Box 4.3). Following a significant exposure, baseline and six month blood samples are taken from the HCW to establish that transmission of infection has not occurred. Blood samples are retained for two years.

MANAGEMENT OF HEPATITIS C EXPOSURES

At the present time there is no effective prophylaxis or vaccine available against hepatitis C. Most sharps exposures are likely to involve patients who are chronic carriers of the disease as up to 85% of HCV infections are asymptomatic. Only HCV RNA-positive patients pose a risk for HCV transmission.

Box 4.2 Basic assessment of patient risk factors for BBV exposure*

- Has the patient ever had HCV, HBV or HIV infection?
- If the patient has HIV, are they taking anti-retroviral drugs, is their viral status known and verified?
- Engaged in unprotected sex between men (MSM)?
- Shared injecting equipment when using recreational drugs, performance- or image-enhancing drugs?
- Had unprotected sex in a high-prevalence country (>2%) or with a person from a high-prevalence country/risk group (e.g. MSM, sex worker), e.g. Africa, Central, East and South-east Asia, etc.?
- Received a blood transfusion in the UK before 1991 or at any time in a country with a high prevalence of BBV infection?
- Had unprotected sexual intercourse with any of the above?

* Occupational health service will advise on in-depth risk assessment and sexual history.

Box 4.3 Information required to assess the exposure risk to BBVs

Healthcare personnel's immune status for hepatitis B
Postvaccination hepatitis, HBs antibody titre:
- Good responders anti-HBs level of >100 IU/mL
- Poor responders anti-HBs level of >10 IU/mL but <100 IU/mL
- Non-responders anti-HBs level of <10 IU/mL
Date of administration of hepatitis B vaccination or booster inoculation

Assessment of injury: factors that increase risk of BBV transmission
Percutaneous needlestick injury > mucocutaneous exposure (broken skin, abrasions, cuts, eczema, etc.) or exposure of mucous membrane including the eye (splash)
Visible blood on the device that caused the injury
Source blood containing a high viral load

Risks associated with HIV transmission
A deep penetrating injury
Needle placed directly in an artery or vein
Blood visible in the LA cartridge of an aspirating syringe
Exposure to large volumes of blood
A detectable viral load in an HIV-positive source patient currently on cART, untreated HIV-positive patient or diagnosed with AIDS

Protocols for hepatitis C testing of healthcare personnel exposed to a known HCV-positive source are as follows.

- Initial baseline antibody test to HCV (to determine if the healthcare worker is an existing carrier of HCV).
- Obtain serum/EDTA for genome 1 detection at six and 12 weeks.
- Obtain serum for anti-HCV antibodies at 12 and 24 weeks.
- If antibody positive then a confirmatory HCV RNA detection test (polymerase chain reaction) is performed.
- If the individual is going to receive antiviral treatment, then genotyping, viral load estimate and liver function tests (LFTs) are undertaken.

If the source of the blood is unknown then the recipient's antibody levels are retested at six months, which allows time for viral incubation and antibody formation to occur. The subsequent results will inform the decision on whether or not to commence antiviral therapy. There is usually no need to stop performing invasive dental procedures whilst waiting for the test results. Epidemiological surveys have shown that risk of transmission of infection from a healthcare worker to a patient during an invasive procedure is small if standard precautions are followed.

POSTEXPOSURE PROPHYLAXIS FOR HIV AND HEPATITIS B

After a sharps injury, studies indicate that there may be a 'window of opportunity' to avert HIV or HBV infection by inhibiting viral replication following an exposure. Once HIV crosses a mucosal barrier, it may take up to 48–72 hours before HIV can be detected within regional lymph nodes and up to five days before it can be detected in blood. Initiation of combination antiretroviral therapy (cART) has been shown to reduce dissemination and replication of HIV virus in all tissues if initiated early after inoculation in animal studies. Inhibition of HBV viral replication is achieved by stimulation of the protective immune response to hepatitis B with a HBV vaccine or anti-HBV immunoglobulin.

HIV postexposure prophylaxis (PEP) is prescribed based on a case-by-case risk assessment undertaken by the physician in conjunction with the wishes of the staff member. PEP will not normally be offered if the source case is HIV negative or following a risk assessment that indicates the risk of HIV infection is unlikely. In the UK, HIV PEP is no longer recommended if the source patient is on effective cART with a confirmed and sustained (>6 months) undetectable plasma HIV viral load. The dates and results of the source's last viral load tests should be verified with their clinic for a minimum of the last six months, and recorded in the PEP assessment. If there is any doubt about the source's viral load or adherence to cART then PEP should be given as a precaution following occupational exposure. However, the healthcare worker can request HIV PEP should they wish to do so. Note that blood from an HIV-positive source coming into contact with intact skin is not a transmission risk. In some countries, HIV PEP is offered after all occupational percutaneous exposure injuries and mucosal exposures to blood when the HIV status of the source is positive or unknown.

To achieve optimal efficiency with HIV PEP, it should be initiated as soon as possible after the exposure (e.g. within 1–2 hours), but can be offered up to 72 hours later. A typical HIV PEP regimen would include a combination of antiviral drugs, e.g. raltegravir/Truvada® for 28 days. Guidance on the most appropriate regimen is updated regularly and country variations may be in force locally. cART drug combinations may be adapted to take into account antiretroviral drug resistance in the source patient or drug interactions in the recipient. A full course of treatment lasts for 28 days, but it can be stopped early if the patient is found to be HIV negative on blood tests. Follow-up HIV testing is recommended at 12 weeks and the recipient is monitored for symptoms of a seroconversion illness, such as flu-like illness and skin rash. A postexposure regimen to prevent hepatitis B infection is outlined in Box 4.4.

Box 4.4 HBV postexposure prophylaxis regimen

- Hepatitis B vaccine is highly effective at preventing infection if given shortly after exposure.
- Ideally, immunization should commence within 48 hours, although it should still be considered up to a week after exposure.
- The vaccine is not effective in patients with acute hepatitis B and is not necessary for individuals known to have markers of current (HBsAg) or past (anti-HB) infection. However, immunization should not be delayed whilst waiting for test results.

Specific hepatitis B immunoglobulin (HBIG)
- Use of HBIG *in addition* to hepatitis B vaccine is recommended only in high-risk situations or in a known non-responder to hepatitis B vaccine.
- Gives *immediate but temporary protection* after accidental inoculation or contamination with hepatitis B-infected blood. It will not affect the development of vaccine-induced long-term active immunity.
- HBIG should be given as soon as possible; ideally it is given concurrently with the first dose of hepatitis B vaccine but at a different site.
- HBIG should be considered up to a week after exposure as although virus multiplication may not be completely inhibited at this stage, it may prevent severe illness and development of a chronic carrier state.
- At six months, the person is monitored for symptoms of a seroconversion illness.

If a dental student or a member of the dental team becomes infected with hepatitis B or C, then specialist occupational advice must be sought as they may be prohibited from providing exposure-prone dental treatment in accordance with national guidelines. HIV seropositive students and dental personnel can now continue to perform EPPs in the UK and in many other countries (see Chapter 3).

RECORDING OF SHARPS INJURIES

All sharps injuries and significant splashes, however minor, must be recorded in an accident logbook. Include a full description of the incident, who was involved (both patient and staff member) and how it was managed. Data protection regulations require that confidentiality is maintained and the information stored securely (e.g. in a lockable, fire-retardant filing cabinet) and retained for a minimum of three years. Therefore, accidents must be recorded on separate forms marked with an identification system for chronological record keeping. Accident records may be required for future insurance or benefits claims and provide contemporaneous evidence of a specific occupational exposure. In the UK, in the event of a member of the dental team developing HIV infection or hepatitis B or C following an incident in the workplace, the employer must report the incident to the Health and Safety Executive under the Reporting of Injuries, Diseases and Dangerous Occurrences (RIDDOR) Regulations 2013. Sharps incidents with a sharp known to be contaminated with a BBV are reported as a 'dangerous occurrence'.

CLINICAL GOVERNANCE AND ACCIDENT RISK ASSESSMENT

Reviewing clinical procedures for preventing sharps injuries and undertaking risk assessments are important components of clinical governance and a requirement of the Health and Safety (Sharp Instruments in Healthcare) Regulations and COSHH Regulations. So do not 'waste' accidents and near misses; use them for staff training. It is important that the dentist creates an environment in which team members feel confident to inform them that something might go wrong or has already done so. The circumstances that lead up to the incident should be identified and analysed and appropriate steps taken to prevent a future recurrence of the incident.

REFERENCES AND WEBSITES

Expert Advisory Group on AIDS (EAGA). EAGA Guidance on HIV Post-Exposure Prophylaxis. Available at: www.gov.uk/government/publications/eaga-guidance-on-hiv-post-exposure-prophylaxis (accessed 28 October 2016).

Hadler SC, Sorley DL, Acree KH *et al.* (1981) An outbreak of hepatitis B in a dental practice. *Annals of Internal Medicine*, **95**, 133–138.

Health & Safety Executive (2013) Health and Safety (Sharp Instruments in Healthcare) Regulations, Guidance for Employers and Employees. Available at: www.hse.gov.uk/pubns/hsis7.pdf (accessed 28 October 2016).

Woode OM, Wellington E, Rice B *et al.* (2014) Bloodborne Viruses: Eye of the Needle. Available at: www.gov.uk/government/publications/bloodborne-viruses-eye-of-the-needle (accessed 28 October 2016).

Young TN, Arens FJ, Kennedy GE, Laurie JW, Rutherford GW. (2007) Antiretroviral post-exposure prophylaxis (PEP) for occupational HIV exposure. *Cochrane Database of Systematic Reviews*, **1**, CD002835.

Zakrzewska JM, Greenwood I, Jackson J. (2001) Introducing safety syringes into a UK dental school – a controlled study. *British Dental Journal*, **190**, 88–92.

Chapter 5

Hand hygiene

HANDS AS A SOURCE OF INFECTION

Microbial colonization of the hands

The entire surface of the human body is colonized by micro-organisms. High bacterial counts in the region of a million colony-forming bacteria are found on the skin below the waist, particularly in the warm moist perineal and inguinal areas. Lower numbers of bacteria colonize the skin of the hands, trunk and underarms. Skin colonization increases dramatically in chronic skin conditions, such as dermatitis or acne. Most people shed about a million skin scales (squames) per day. Attached to the shed skin scales are micro-organisms, mainly desiccation-resistant species such as staphylococci and enterococci. The shed bacteria are deposited on clothes, uniforms, masks and in the surrounding local environment.

Resident and transient bacteria

Skin of the hands harbours two main types of microorganisms, resident and transient, which colonize and survive on the hands for differing amounts of time. Resident flora found on the hands include mainly Gram-positive, low virulence micro-organisms that are rarely transmitted by hand contact and are not easily removed through hand hygiene. The transient hand flora consists mainly of Gram-negative bacteria that are an important cause of nosocomial infections that can be removed by hand hygiene.

Resident micro-organisms, as their name suggests, make up the persistent microbial flora of the hands living on the surface and within the superficial

Basic Guide to Infection Prevention and Control in Dentistry, Second Edition.
Caroline L. Pankhurst.
© 2017 John Wiley & Sons Ltd. Published 2017 by John Wiley & Sons Ltd.
Companion website: www.wiley.com/go/pankhurst/infection-prevention

structures of the skin without causing infection. For most of the time, the bacterial relationship with the host is symbiotic. However, if the intact skin is breached by surgical interventions such as suturing then resident species (e.g. *Staphylococcus epidermidis*) can become opportunistic pathogens causing wound or deep-seated infections. Transient micro-organisms that include environmental and pathogenic bacteria, fungi or viruses colonize the skin for short periods of time, usually only hours or days.

Following even brief episodes of personal contact, such as shaking hands or touching a patient's face, hundreds or thousands of bacteria are transferred onto the dental healthcare personnel's hands. Not surprisingly, even higher rates of bacterial transfer can occur during patient treatment, as hands become progressively colonized with organisms from the respiratory tract and mouth. After the initial contamination of the skin, the rapidly dividing bacteria are transferred to previously uncontaminated parts of the hands, wrists or cuffs as the latter brush over the hands. Bacterial replication will continue in a linear fashion over time until the hands are cleaned. It is thus easy inadvertently to transfer the patient's pathogenic microbes growing on your hands by touch and inoculate your own mouth and eyes with pathogens.

Direct contact via hands is the major route of spread for a number of organisms including MRSA, influenza viruses, herpes simplex (the cause of cold sores) and herpes zoster viruses (the cause of shingles; see Chapter 2). The main purpose of hand hygiene is to remove or destroy the transient flora acquired through contact with patients and their surroundings or contaminated equipment, as well as the physical removal of dirt, blood and body fluids.

HANDS AS A SOURCE OF HOSPITAL-ACQUIRED INFECTION

> Hands form a link in the chain of infection.

Hands of healthcare workers and patients are instrumental in the spread of multidrug-resistant bacteria such as MRSA and *Clostridium difficile*. About 5–10% of patients during their hospital stay will pick up a healthcare-associated infection (HCAI). Some of these infections may have fatal consequences, but all will add to the cost of patient treatment and length of hospital stay, and cause unnecessary suffering and inconvenience to the patient and their family and friends. In the USA annually, 2 000 000 patients become seriously ill as a result of acquiring an infection in hospital, with approximately 80 000 deaths. It is estimated that 600 000 of these HCAIs are due to HCWs failing to wash their hands before and after every patient contact. In England, healthcare-associated infection costs in the region of £3–8000 per infection. Yet this unwelcome chain of events can be broken simply and expediently by effective use of hand hygiene. Results from the data collected over the last 30 plus years provide strong evidence that hand hygiene is the single most important method of reducing cross-transmission of infectious organisms (Loveday et al., 2014).

When to clean your hands

The World Health Organization (WHO) actively promotes the concept of 'five moments for hand hygiene'. The five moments are based on the scientific evidence for the risks of transmission of microbes by hands and the opportunities for effective hand hygiene to prevent transmission. This approach recommends healthcare workers to clean their hands:

1. before touching a patient
2. before clean/aseptic procedures
3. after body fluid exposure/risk, e.g. saliva, blood or other bodily fluid
4. after touching a patient
5. after touching patient surroundings.

This simple but effective concept has been adopted worldwide as a framework for use in national campaigns to promote hand hygiene practice through the action of training, audit with feedback and as a base for national policies.

It is very easy to contaminate inanimate objects in the surgery unthinkingly by touching them with gloved hands during patient treatment. At particular risk from hand and environmental contamination are computer keyboard and mouse, pens and patient's notes. In hospital studies nearly all patients' case notes were contaminated with pathogenic bacteria, including MRSA. Reception staff and others are advised to clean their hands after touching notes or surfaces in close proximity to patients (Figure 5.1).

HAND HYGIENE AND TEAMWORKING

The initial impetus for the WHO campaign to promote hand hygiene was the compelling results obtained from the longitudinal study undertaken in hospitals in Geneva, Switzerland, by Pittet et al. (2000). In the study, alcohol/chlorhexidine gluconate 0.5% hand rub solution was introduced as the focal point of a hospital-wide hand hygiene campaign. With the co-operation of the hospital staff, their campaign achieved an impressive 44% reduction in HCAIs and a 50% fall in patient colonization with MRSA. Many more recent studies have confirmed their findings. An important lesson was learnt from their work that is of direct relevance to dentistry. Long-term success (the study was conducted over

(a) (b)

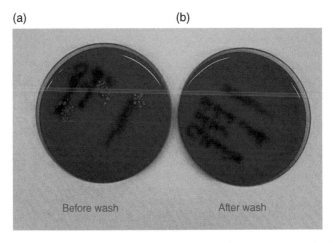

Before wash   After wash

Figure 5.1 Microbiological hand sampling before (a) and after (b) cleaning with alcohol based hand rub.

six years) was dependent on the active involvement of senior personnel who were publically seen to endorse the campaign. Posters and other promotional material reinforced the main message of the campaign. Staff received regular feedback from local audits evaluating their compliance with hand hygiene measures, which improved staff motivation. Similarly, dentists and infection control leads as team leaders can influence the behaviour of other members of the dental team by acting as positive role models. Staff are more likely to follow suit and embrace prevention protocols if dentists or, in the case of dental schools, professors are witnessed to actively comply with infection control measures.

Choosing the correct hand hygiene product

The term 'hand hygiene' encompasses traditional hand washing with soap and water or antiseptic hand washes and the newer technique of hand rubbing with disinfectant, alcohol-based hand rubs (ABHR) that do not require running water. Hand rubs are sometimes referred to as 'leave-on products' as they are not rinsed off after use. ABHRs are formulated as gels, rinses and foams.

Not all skin-cleaning agents are equally effective at removing organic material or killing microbes (Table 5.1). Consequently, choosing the most appropriate agent for hand hygiene will depend on when and why the hands are being cleaned. Hand hygiene is used in three circumstances: hand washing (social hand hygiene), hand disinfection using an ABHR (hygienic hand hygiene) and surgical scrub (surgical hand hygiene) (Table 5.2). It is impossible to completely sterilise the hands as resident bacteria survive in the deep skin hair follicles and sebaceous glands, but if hands are cleaned effectively only very low numbers of bacteria will remain (see Table 5.1).

HAND HYGIENE

Table 5.1 Comparison of the properties of common hand hygiene products

Type of hand-cleaning agent	Action	Inhibited by organic material	Active against *C. difficile*	Limitations	Type of hand hygiene
Chlorhexidine and Triclosan	Rapid Binds to skin; remains active for up to 6 hours	No	Yes	Chlorhexidine may cause irritant/ allergic dermatitis in some people*	Hygienic Surgical
Iodophors	Rapid	Yes	Yes	Inhibited by organic material. May cause skin irritation in some people. Staining of skin	Surgical
Alcohol-based hand rubs and gels	Very rapid Short-lived	Yes	No	Inhibited by organic material, e.g. blood	Hygienic Surgical

* Chlorhexidine can trigger anaphylaxis in allergic individuals.

Alcohol-based hand rubs

Alcohol-based hand rubs are recommended for hand disinfection by the WHO.

Alcohol-based hand rubs were originally promoted by healthcare campaigners to encourage improved compliance and overcome perceived and real barriers to hand washing. In surveys, conventional detergents and soaps were shunned by healthcare personnel as being damaging to the skin. Inconveniently located sinks, demanding workload, tiredness and time constraints were also cited as reasons not to wash hands. Most hand rubs have the advantage of containing an emollient to protect the skin, are inexpensive and hand hygiene can be performed at the chair-side. Hand rubs are available in an individual dispenser that can be carried in the pocket or on a belt and are ideal where there is limited access to a sink, such as on a domiciliary visit.

Commercial disinfectant hand rubs come in a wide variety of formulations. Typically, the active ingredients comprise an alcoholic solution ranging from 65% to 75% with either a low or high concentration of detergents, disinfectants and surfactants such as biguanides, quaternary ammonium compounds or peroxides. Commercial products that contain predominantly ethanol are diluted from 10% to 40% by weight with water to enhance denaturation of

Table 5.2 The three types of hand hygiene

Type	Product	Duration (entire procedure)	Purpose
Hand washing	Soap and water	40–60 seconds	Removal of dirt, body fluids and transient micro-organisms
Hand disinfection	Alcohol-based hand rub	20–30 seconds	Killing and removal of transient microbes and reduction of resident flora
Surgical scrub	Aqueous antimicrobial disinfectant Alcohol-based hand rub	2 minutes	Killing and removal of transient micro-organisms and substantially reduction of resident micro-organisms

microbial proteins. Alcohols in the form of ethanol or isopropyl alcohol demonstrate rapid action against a wide range of Gram-positive and Gram-negative species, including MRSA and vancomycin-resistant enterococci. Alcohol's reactive hydroxyl (-OH) group readily forms hydrogen bonds with proteins, which leads to loss of structure and function, causing protein and other macromolecules to precipitate. Alcohol also lyses the bacterial cytoplasmic membrane, which releases the cellular contents and leads to bacterial inactivation. As little as 15 seconds of vigorous alcohol-based hand rubbing has been shown to be effective in preventing transmission of Gram-negative bacteria (GNB) and kills 98% of the GNB (Figure 5.2). However, most manufacturers and the WHO recommend cleaning the hands for a period of 30 seconds. Allowing time for the alcohol to completely evaporate from hands is essential for microbial killing. Because of alcohol's rapid speed of action and multiple, non-specific toxic effects, microbes are rarely able to develop resistance to alcohol. As alcohols evaporate, no significant antiseptic residue is left on the skin that could contribute to the development of microbial resistance, whereas concerns have been raised regarding the detergent component of hand rubs. Gram-negative bacteria have developed resistance to a range of detergents used in healthcare with the likelihood in some instances of co-selection of antibiotic resistance.

Limitations of alcohol-based hand rubs

Use alcohol-based hand rub only on visibly clean hands.

Hand rubs have limitations which need to be recognized if they are to be used safely. ABHRs are specifically designed to promote the frequency of hand

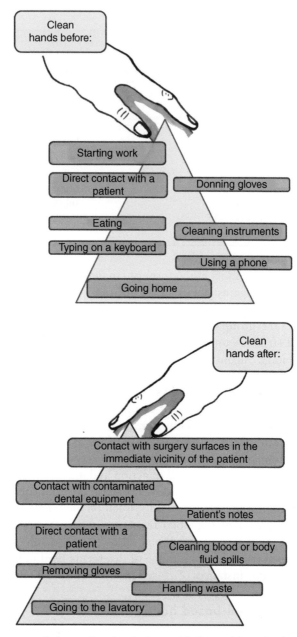

Figure 5.2 Summary of when to clean hands. Figure a) before and figure b) after the listed activity. Illustration by Georgia Sweet.

hygiene at busy times. Their deceptive ease of use can lead to tokenistic, cursory decontamination of the hands, especially when there is a heavy workload or at the end of working day. ABHRs are unsuitable when hands are visibly soiled with organic material such as blood or dirt. Importantly, they are ineffective against spore-forming bacteria such as *C. difficile* and noroviruses that cause acute gastroenteritis (known colloquially as 'winter vomiting bug'). Paradoxically, recent over-reliance on ABHRs and the concomitant reduction in traditional hand washing with soaps and antiseptic hand washes may have contributed to the increased incidence of *C. difficile* diarrhoeal infections observed in the UK. In contrast, against other microbes (e.g. rhinoviruses), ABHRs are more effective than soap and water.

Unlike chlorhexidine or Triclosan, which bind to the skin and can remain active for up to six hours, their action is short-lived. The alcohol component evaporates rapidly, often before the user has been able to spread the solution over all parts of their hands, so areas escape exposure to the bactericidal action of the alcohol. Gels and foam formulations overcome this problem by slowing down evaporation, increasing the active contact time and thereby enhancing bacterial killing. The emollient added to hand rubs and gels can build up on hands, giving a feeling of greasiness which some people find distasteful. Excess emollient is also transferred from the hands to clinic surfaces, contaminating them. To avoid these problems, hands should be washed with plain soap and water at intervals throughout the day.

Systemic effects of hand rubs

Recent data have shown systemic exposure with repetitive long-term use of both Triclosan and alcohol-based rubs on hands. Triclosan and triclocarban can cause alterations in thyroid and reproductive systems of neonatal and adolescent animals. Studies in humans have shown detectable blood alcohol levels after use of alcohol-containing hand rubs or surgical hand rubs. Alcohol absorption through human skin is less effective than absorption via the oral route, the more normal route for imbibing alcoholic drinks. Based on the available data, on moderate hand rub use (7.5–40 ABHR applications per hour), the highest observed exposure was 1500 mg of alcohol, equivalent to 10% of an alcohol-containing drink. Overall, the exposure is low during a typical working day in dentistry. As always, there is a risk versus benefit balance for products used in healthcare and the value of effective hand hygiene in infection prevention and control cannot be overstated. In the USA, the Food and Drug Administration (FDA) is actively monitoring both animal and human pharmacokinetic studies evaluating antiseptic ingredients used in rubs and washes, in order to identify any potential safety concerns and help determine the safety margins applicable to healthcare use.

Storage of alcohol-based hand rub

Alcohol-based hand rubs are flammable and have a low flashpoint and can be ignited by static electricity. Care should be taken to avoid splashing near an open flame or contact with direct heat or sunlight, especially when ABHRs are stored in bulk. Fortunately, the numbers of fires directly attributable to combustion of ABHR are few. As is the case with all disinfectants, a Control of Substances Hazardous to Health (COSHH) safety assessment is required. Try to keep ABHRs out of reach of curious children who might be tempted to drink them. Avoiding the use of the term 'alcohol' in signs and patient information literature will help to dissuade desperate patients from taking a surreptitious swig! In the UK, deaths from acute alcohol poisoning caused by drinking ABHRs acquired from hospitals have been reported in homeless adults.

HAND HYGIENE TECHNIQUE

Remove rings and watches

Microbiological studies have shown that the skin under rings becomes heavily colonized with bacteria, such as *Staphylococcus aureus* and Gram-negative species. The same bacterial species were found to persist for months under a ring and may triple the risk of GNB carriage. Fewer bacteria are found under silver than gold and platinum rings, as silver is inhibitory to the growth of bacteria. Rings and watches may also prevent effective cleaning of the skin because the wearer does not want to damage a precious item of jewellery or dislodge a gemstone and so avoids cleaning their hands effectively. Therefore, it is recommended that watches and rings (except for plain wedding bands) are removed before the start of the treatment session. Moreover, gloves are more prone to tear when rings are worn on the hand. Artificial nails and chipped nail polish also harbour bacteria and *Candida* spp. and have been implicated as the source of outbreaks of bacterial and fungal infections amongst patients in hospital wards. Artificial fingernails became colonised with GNB more frequently than natural nails and alcohol-based hand rubs were less effective in eliminating GNB from artificial nails. Hence, it is best to keep fingernails short, clean and free from nail polish and artificial nails.

Standard hand hygiene technique

The standard hand-washing technique is versatile and appropriate for all types of hand hygiene. It can be used to apply soap, aqueous antimicrobial hand wash and ABHRs to the hands.

At the start of a treatment session, hands should be washed with soap and water and thereafter with hand rub. There is a science to hand washing/

rubbing just as there is to cleaning teeth effectively. Employing a standardized method ensures that all surfaces of the hands and wrists are exposed to the disinfectant and thoroughly cleaned in a systematic manner (Figure 5.3). The sequence of hand movements is formulated to concentrate on the heavily contaminated fingertips and areas of the hand that are commonly missed – finger and thumb webs, cuticles, wrists and backs of hands as shown in Figure 5.4. None of the disinfectants used in antimicrobial soaps are particularly effective at killing spore-forming bacteria. It is now appreciated that removal of spores

(a)

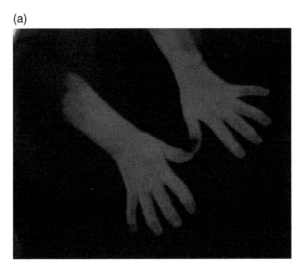

(b)

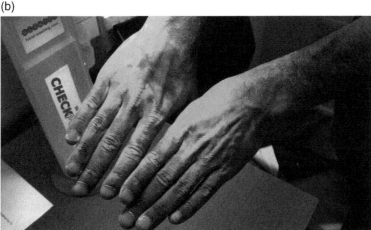

Figure 5.3 (a) Correct dispersal of hand rub. Blue fluorescent UV alcohol-based hand rub is applied to all parts of the hands and wrists before cleaning them. (b) Failure to distribute a green fluorescent hand rub to all parts of the hands, showing a typical pattern where the dorsum of the hands is missed. Microbes are only killed where the rub makes contact with the skin.

(a)

(b)

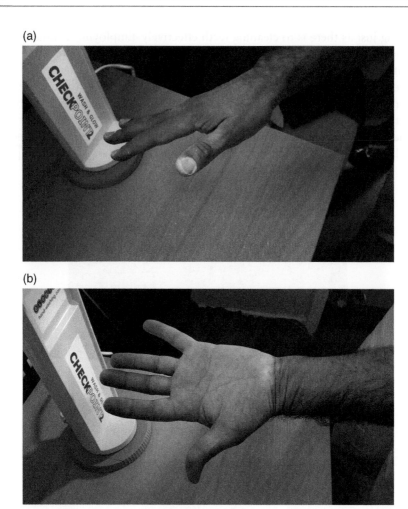

Figure 5.4 Commonly missed areas when cleaning hands. Hands and wrists inspected under UV light after cleaning hands with a green fluorescent UV-sensitive alcohol-based hand rub. Areas of hands that are missed still glow under the UV light. (a) Thumb, thumb web and cuticles. (b) Wrist.

from the hands requires the physical action of vigorous rubbing and rinsing under running water. The final stage is thoroughly drying the hands. This helps to maintain skin integrity and prevent onward transmission of microbes, which can proliferate on damp hands and damaged skin. Moist hands transfer a significantly higher number of microbes to hard surfaces and fabrics than hands that are carefully dried. Hand hygiene is demonstrated on a video available on the companion website.

When using the standard technique (Figure 5.5) with ABHRs, it is important to use a sufficient quantity of the rub to completely cover all surfaces of the

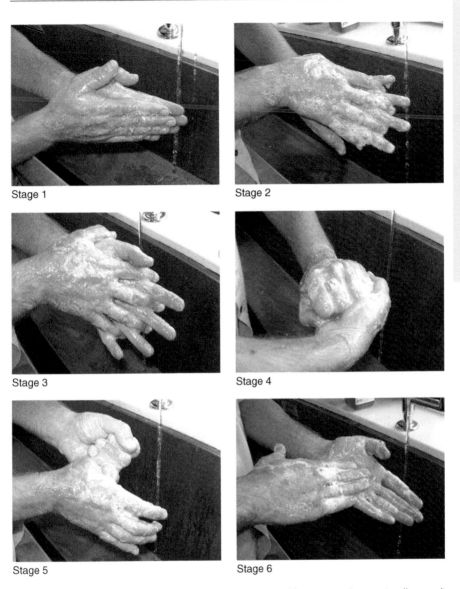

Stage 1

Stage 2

Stage 3

Stage 4

Stage 5

Stage 6

Figure 5.5 Standard hand hygiene technique. Can be used for soap and water (as illustrated) or for applying alcohol-based hand rubs. The initial wetting of the hands with water and the final drying of the hands is not illustrated. Source: Photos kindly supplied by Paul Morris, Queen's University, Belfast.

hands and wrists. The WHO has recommended filling the well created in a cupped palm of hand with approximately 3.5 mL of rub solution equivalent to 2–3 aliquots of dispensed solution, then vigorously cleaning hands and wrists for 30 seconds.

Good practice guidance for hand hygiene

- A poster showing hand-washing protocol should be displayed in the surgery.
- Cuts and abrasions less than 24 hours old must be covered with a waterproof dressing. After 24 hours, the body's natural defences 'seal' small cuts and wounds.
- Fingernails should be kept short, clean and free from nail polish, artificial nails and nail art.
- Wristwatches and jewellery should be removed, and any long-sleeved clothing be rolled up/removed. Rings (except plain wedding rings) should not be worn during a clinical session. Manipulate wedding ring when washing hands so that cleaning solution can contact skin under the ring or preferably remove it before hand hygiene.
- Hand cream should be applied regularly throughout the day to protect skin from drying. However, communal tubs should be avoided as these can become contaminated.

Hand hygiene technique: hand washing

Hand washing with liquid soap or aqueous antimicrobial hand wash solutions.

- Washing procedure takes approximately 40–60 seconds.
- Wet hands under lukewarm running water before applying liquid soap or antiseptic hand wash solution into cupped hands. Use enough soap/antiseptic solution to cover the hands completely.
- Rub hands together vigorously to lather all surfaces of hands and wrists.
- Wash palms, backs of hands, finger and thumb webs, tips of fingers and thumbs, especially the nail area (see Figure 5.4).
- Rinse hands thoroughly under running water.
- Dry hands completely with a soft, absorbent single-use disposable paper towel. Air and jet driers are not appropriate for use in clinical areas.

Hand hygiene technique using an alcohol-based hand rub

- Fill the well of a cupped hand with alcohol-based solution (approximately 2–3 dispensed aliquots).
- Distribute solution evenly over every part of the hands and wrists.
- Rub hands together vigorously using the standard method for 20–30 seconds. Pay particular attention to the tips, webs and nailbeds of the fingers and thumbs.
- Continue until the solution has completely evaporated and the hands are dry.

Surgical hand hygiene

For surgical procedures (e.g. minor oral surgery, periodontal and implant surgery), more extensive disinfection, referred to as antisepsis or surgical scrub of the hands and arms, is required. This is in order to reduce the numbers of resident bacteria to a minimum, although it is not possible to sterilise the skin. First, wash the hands, nails and forearms with an antimicrobial disinfectant hand wash solution marketed as a surgical scrub for two minutes, followed by thorough rinsing and drying of the skin. Although the term 'scrub' is retained, the use of nailbrushes on skin and nails and nail picks does not decrease bacterial numbers and is unnecessary.

Alternatively, use an ABHR. Prewash hands, nails and forearms with a mild neutral soap and water followed by two sequential 5 mL applications of alcohol hand rub gel. Vigorously rub hands and forearms with the solution for two minutes, using the standard method described above. Comparative experiments have shown that the two-stage technique with alcohol hand rubs is as effective as conventional hand scrubbing with an aqueous antimicrobial disinfectant hand wash solution. By using either method, the bacterial count on the hands will remain sufficiently low throughout a six-hour surgical procedure.

Consumables and facilities for hand hygiene area

- Handwash sink and surrounds should be visibly clean and free of clutter.
- The hand wash sink should be easily accessible and must be dedicated for hand washing only. The sink should have no overflows or plugs in order to prevent contamination of the taps with *Pseudomonas* spp. (see Chapter 9).
- Taps should preferably be sensor, elbow-, or foot-operated lever taps to reduce the risk of hand contamination and be fitted with thermal mixer valves both to avoid scalding of the hands and to prevent contamination of the tap by legionellae (see Chapter 9).
- To reduce formation of contaminated aerosols and to prevent indirect contamination of the taps, the water jet should not flow directly into the plughole (see Chapter 8).
- A choice of wall-mounted dispensers of liquid soap, aqueous detergent and ABHR should be provided. ABHR dispensers should be sited away from the other dispensers to avoid any confusion with wash-off products.
- Hand hygiene solutions should be dispensed in disposable rather than refillable cartridges/bottles. Refillable dispensers are likely to become contaminated with micro-organisms during the 'topping up' process and therefore should be avoided. Keep the dispenser nozzle clean.
- Soap bars are not suitable for use in the clinical setting as they easily become colonized with Gram-negative bacteria and *Pseudomonas* spp. and act as a source of cross-infection.

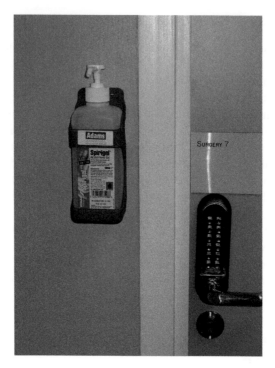

Figure 5.6 Wall-mounted alcohol-based hand rub at the entrance to the surgery for use by patients and staff.

- Wall-mounted disposable paper towels should be used. Reusable towels are not suitable for clinical settings as they become readily contaminated with micro-organisms. Dispose of the used towels in foot-operated waste bins to avoid using the hands to raise the lid of the waste bin.
- Nailbrushes are *not* indicated for hand hygiene in dental practice. If nails need to be cleaned before surgery, then a sterile brush should be used on each occasion.
- Patients on entering and exiting the treatment area should be encouraged to clean their hands with alcohol-based hand rub/gel, as they are potentially part of the chain of infection. This is particularly relevant when patients have been coughing or sneezing. Therefore consider placing a wall-mounted dispenser of hand rub solution in the patient waiting room and/or at the entrance to the surgery (Figure 5.6).

HAND CARE AND PREVENTION OF DERMATITIS

The keratin-rich layers of intact skin form a natural barrier to infection. Hence it is essential that you protect your hands from damage by wearing heavy-duty gloves for work in the home and garden. Sebum from the sebaceous glands helps to maintain skin integrity. Skin pH is mildly acidic, therefore regular use of alkaline soaps and disinfectants can alter the pH and cause drying and abrasion of the hands, which in some people can result in irritant dermatitis. Alcohols are inherently drying. Products containing 70% alcohol by weight cause the least dehydration of the skin and are the most popular with users. To compensate for the dehydrating effect, manufacturers add emollients, which is why these products cause fewer abrasions, drying and irritation to the hands than soaps or disinfectant washes.

Members of the dental team or students who have an existing skin condition such as dermatitis or who develop skin irritation while using particular products such as gloves or disinfectants should seek expert dermatological advice on treatment and management. Allergenicity is routinely reported with antimicrobial detergent solutions; the latter may also cause drying and abrasion of the skin on repeated use, whereas alcohol has a low allergenic potential. However, as may occur with any skin preparation, a small proportion of people do develop hypersensitivity to alcohol-based hand rubs. Allergic reactions and cases of contact dermatitis are usually in response to the other added ingredients. Affected healthcare personnel should change to an alternative product and seek medical advice from their local occupational health physician or general medical practitioner.

Protective effect of emollient hand creams

Emollient hand cream applied several times a day helps to prevent skin problems from developing. Shared communal pots of hand cream rapidly become contaminated, so either individual supplies or elbow-operated pump dispensers

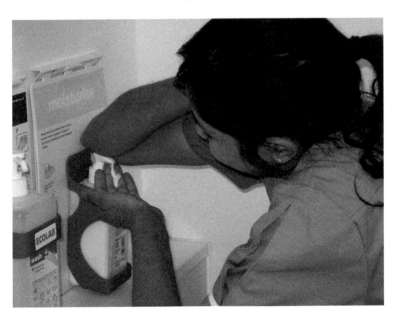

Figure 5.7 Wall-mounted elbow-operated emollient hand cream dispenser.

of hand cream are advised (Figure 5.7). Petroleum-based hand creams are not recommended as they can adversely affect latex, thereby increasing glove permeability, which in turn permits ingress of micro-organisms. Furthermore, hand cream has been demonstrated to reduce cross-transmission by preventing excess shedding of residential bacteria from dry, flaky skin.

REFERENCES AND WEBSITES

Health Protection Scotland (2015) National Infection Prevention and Control Manual. Available at: www.hps.scot.nhs.uk/haiic/ic/guidelinedetail.aspx?id=49785# (accessed 30 October 2016).

Loveday HP, Wilson JA, Pratta RJ *et al.* (2014) Epic3: national evidence-based guidelines for preventing healthcare-associated infections in NHS hospitals in England. *Journal of Hospital Infection*, **86**(Suppl. 1), S1–S70.

Pittet D, Hugonnet S, Mourouga P *et al.* (2000) Effectiveness of a hospital-wide programme to improve compliance with hand hygiene. *Lancet*, **356**, 1307–12.

World Health Organization (2009) WHO Guidelines on Hand Hygiene in Healthcare. Available at: www.who.int/gpsc/5may/tools/9789241597906/en/(accessed 30 October 2016).

Chapter 6

Personal protection for prevention of cross-infection

WHY WE WEAR PERSONAL PROTECTIVE EQUIPMENT

During the working day, our clothing and uniforms become progressively more contaminated by nosocomial pathogens (micro-organisms in the clinical environment) which can become a source of cross-infection. Nosocomial microbes account for two-thirds of micro-organisms found on clothing and our own skin flora shed on dead skin cells comprises the remaining third. Areas of the body that are particularly heavily colonized with microbes are areas exposed to splatter such as forearm, upper chest and face and those parts most frequently touched by our hands, i.e. below the waist, sleeves and pockets. During dental treatment, other items worn by the dental team, such as badges and lanyards, jewellery and even mobile phones kept in a pocket, become contaminated. Wearing a plastic apron or gown forms a physical barrier and significantly reduces contamination of workwear. We also need to protect vulnerable parts of the body from contamination, for example the mucous membranes of the eyes, nose, mouth and lungs as well as damaged or broken skin. This is the reason why infection control policies require the dental team to wear personal protective equipment (PPE) such as plastic aprons, impermeable gowns, goggles, masks and disposable gloves. Most PPE is single use, so when we dispose of the PPE as hazardous infectious waste, we simultaneously dispose of the body fluid splatter and pathogens on the PPE, thereby eliminating the cross-infection risk.

In the UK, the Health and Safety at Work Act 1974 and subsequent legislation place a duty of care on employers to provide a safe working environment for their staff, to provide PPE and to train staff to use it appropriately. Staff and

Basic Guide to Infection Prevention and Control in Dentistry, Second Edition.
Caroline L. Pankhurst.
© 2017 John Wiley & Sons Ltd. Published 2017 by John Wiley & Sons Ltd.
Companion website: www.wiley.com/go/pankhurst/infection-prevention

Table 6.1 Risk management hierarchy. Note PPE is at the bottom of the hierarchy

Hierarchy of infection control procedures for personal protection	Examples
Elimination of the hazard	Single-use instruments
Isolation of the hazard	Safety needles
Work practice controls	Hand hygiene
Work behaviour controls	User disposes of sharps
Administrative controls	Infection control policy
Personal protective equipment	Masks, gloves, aprons

students must ensure their own safety by wearing PPE. Patients expect a HCW to wear PPE, which is seen as altruistic and professional. Selection of the most appropriate PPE must be based on a risk assessment of the associated hazards and likelihood and route of transmission of micro-organisms from the source. The practice's infection control policy should reflect:

- type and duration of the task
- potential for exposure to blood and other body fluids, e.g. respiratory secretions, saliva, vomit
- potential for contamination of non-intact skin or mucous membranes.

Personal protective equipment will function effectively only if selected, worn, removed and discarded correctly. In terms of risk management and according to the law, PPE is considered a 'method of last resort' as PPE is not foolproof and only reduces rather than eliminates the risk (Table 6.1).

Under European law, PPE is classified as a medical device. Therefore, only products carrying the European CE mark should be worn. This denotes that the product fulfils specified performance standards according to the current European legislation.

THE ROLE OF GLOVES

Gloves are single use and should be worn for all routine dental treatment.

When used correctly, wearing gloves:

- protects hands from contamination with blood, saliva and micro-organisms
- reduces the risk of cross-infection
- protects hands from toxic and irritant chemicals

- does not prevent sharps injuries, but the wiping effect of the glove can reduce volume of blood to which the HCW's hand is exposed and in turn the volume inoculated in the event of a percutaneous injury, thereby lowering the risk of transmission of HIV and other blood-borne viruses.

Gloves should be worn during routine dental and surgical treatment, when treating patients, handling waste or mopping up spills. Sterile gloves are worn for invasive surgical procedures. If they are not removed at the end of a task, they become equivalent to 'a second skin', acting as a source of infection. Acquisition and growth dynamics of micro-organisms are similar on bare and gloved hands. But beware –gloves can give a false sense of security to the wearer as gloves do not provide complete protection against hand contamination.

Good practice guide: safe use of gloves in the dental surgery

- Hands must be washed before and after donning gloves. Never consider gloves to be an alternative to hand washing.
- Changing your gloves between patients prevents cross-transmission between patients and contamination of hard surfaces in the surgery. Do not touch patient's notes, pens, computer keyboards, door or drawer handles or your face with gloved hands (see Chapter 8).
- *Never* reuse single-use disposable gloves. There is clinical evidence to demonstrate that glove reuse is associated with transmission of MRSA and Gram-negative bacilli.
- Never wash or disinfect single-use gloves; this reduces the barrier properties and is not a substitute for 'single use'. Note that reuse of any single-use item is in breach of the Medical Devices Regulations (see Chapter 8).
- Keep glove wear to a minimum. Gloves should be applied immediately before starting treatment and removed as soon as the activity is complete.
- Dispose of gloves as hazardous infectious waste.
- Change gloves during very long procedures. After prolonged use, approximately 9–12% of gloves develop perforations or become porous due to hydration of the latex, and may leak. Hepatitis viruses have been transmitted via minor glove perforations.
- Changing your gloves during long procedures reduces excess sweating, which in turn decreases dermal infections or inflammation.
- Remember that hands are not necessarily clean because gloves have been worn. On removing gloves, the patient's micro-organisms can be transmitted from the external surface of the glove to the dentist's hands and need to be removed by hand hygiene.

CHOOSING A SUITABLE GLOVE FOR THE TASK

Natural rubber latex (NRL) gloves and nitrile gloves permit good manual dexterity, are impermeable to microbes and are the most common type of gloves used in healthcare (Table 6.2). Use of nitrile gloves has become very popular in dentistry as a measure to manage the risk of latex allergy occurring in dental students, dental team and patients. However, albeit rarely, allergic responses are also observed when nitrile gloves are worn.

MANAGING AN ALLERGY TO NRL GLOVES

From the mid-1980s onwards, paralleling the routine wearing of gloves in healthcare, the prevalence of latex sensitivity amongst HCWs has risen steadily to 6–18%. Latex sensitivity is particularly common amongst dental students

Table 6.2 Properties of clinical gloves

Type of glove	Properties	Allergies
Natural rubber latex	Impermeable to BBVs, close fitting, do not impair dexterity and are not prone to splitting, resistance to water-based chemicals	Not suitable if allergy to NRL or accelerator
Nitrile (acrylonitrile)	Impermeable to BBVs, close fitting, do not impair dexterity and are not prone to splitting (lowest failure rate under stress conditions), resistance to solvents and oil-based chemicals	Not suitable if allergy to nitrile or accelerator in NRL gloves
Polychloroprene (neoprene)	Impermeable to BBVs	Suitable if allergy to NRL
Vinyl	Impermeable to BBVs and has similar properties to NRL when made to the European Standard. If not, vinyl may be permeable to BBVs, rigid, inflexible and break down in use	Suitable if allergy to NRL/nitrile
Co-polymer (multipolymer synthetic styrene-ethylene-butadine-styrene), e.g. Tactylon®	Similar elasticity and strength to NRL	Contains no NRL proteins and chemicals and is suitable for people with NRL sensitivity
Polythene	Permeable, ill-fitting and prone to splitting and tearing, not suitable for clinical use	Not applicable

BBV, blood-borne virus; NRL, natural rubber latex.

and staff, and can develop even after successfully wearing NRL gloves for many years. Sensitivity is triggered by inhalation of air-borne latex aeroantigens or absorption through damaged skin. NRL is a plant product but other chemicals are added during fabrication of the glove to imbue it with strength, elasticity and flexibility. Varying amounts of NRL and chemical residues may still be present in the glove as a consequence of the manufacturing process. If a latex glove is used then opt for a brand that has low levels of extractable proteins (<50 μg/g of latex proteins) and chemical accelerators (<0.1% w/w of residual accelerators) to minimize the risk of sensitization.

Reactions are classified as:

- *delayed hypersensitivity* (type IV) – resulting in contact dermatitis, rhinitis and conjunctivitis. This is the most common hypersensitivity reaction to NRL or accelerating agents. Response occurs between six and 48 hours after exposure
- *immediate hypersensitivity* (type I) – asthma, urticaria, laryngeal oedema and anaphylactic shock/collapse. Response occurs 15–30 minutes after exposure (Figure 6.1).

Treatment and avoidance strategies are most effective in combating hypersensitivity reactions when initiated early. This relies on recognising the symptoms of immediate and delayed hypersensitivity reactions both in oneself and in patients. If latex sensitivity is suspected, the student, staff member or patient should be referred for specialist advice. Individuals who have experienced a type I reaction to NRL are strongly advised to wear a Medic-Alert bracelet.

Alternatives to NRL gloves that have similar physical properties, i.e. do not impair dexterity and are not prone to splitting and are impermeable to

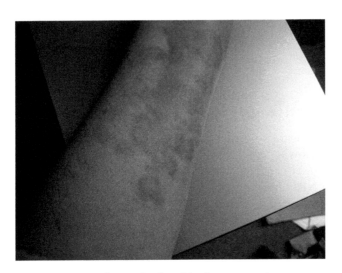

Figure 6.1 Urticarial reaction affecting the skin of the forearm in a dentist.

blood-borne viruses, are shown in Table 6.2. According to health and safety laws in the UK, staff sensitized to NRL gloves must be supplied with appropriate alternatives by their employer. In response to their medico-legal requirements, the majority of dental schools and dental practices have opted to use latex-free gloves and surgery environment as a preventive and safety measure.

Creating a low-latex or latex-free environment

The risk of allergic reactions is triggered not only by latex gloves but also by other latex-containing devices, such as rubber dam, syringe and medication vial bungs, prophylaxis cups, orthodontic elastics, etc. In practices with sensitized individuals, all the dental team may need to change to non-latex gloves due to the generation of aeroallergens in the surgery environment. Susceptible clerical staff who do not have direct contact with patients can also become sensitized as the latex aerosols travel on air currents permeating office areas and waiting rooms. Environmental contamination with latex proteins can be reduced by good ventilation, regular changes of ventilation filters, extensive vacuuming and cleaning of surface contaminated with latex allergens. Equipment in the dental emergency kit should also be free from latex.

MANAGING LATEX ALLERGIES IN PATIENTS

Patients may not always be aware that they have a latex allergy. Individuals who are atopic (predisposition to allergic reactions, such as hay fever, asthma and eczema) are at an increased risk of developing a hypersensitivity reaction to NRL.

Good practice guide: managing latex allergies

- The medical history includes a question on latex allergy (e.g. hypersensitivity reaction following contact with household gloves, blowing up balloons or food allergies to banana, avocado and kiwi fruit which possess shared antigens with NRL).
- If allergy is known, ensure that dental notes are clearly labelled.
- Use latex-free gloves, rubber dams and equipment.
- Remind these patients to inform reception staff when making an appointment and the dentist prior to treatment.

MASKS AND WHEN TO USE THEM

Respiratory protective equipment

Respiratory protective equipment (RPE) is required against organisms that are usually transmitted via the droplet/air-borne route, or when air-borne particles have been artificially created, such as during 'aerosol-generating procedures' (Table 6.3). Two types of masks are used in clinical dentistry as RPE: surgical masks and respirator masks. Note that neither of these masks protects against gases. RPE, like other PPE, should not be relied on for sole protection. To achieve effective protection against respiratory and air-borne pathogens encountered in dentistry, a combination of RPE and safe working practices is required, including rubber dam, high-velocity suction, adequate surgery ventilation, and occupational immunization against infections spread via the respiratory route such as influenza, varicella zoster and measles.

Surgical masks

Fluid-repellent surgical masks act as a physical barrier providing protection to the nose, mouth and upper respiratory tract against sprays, splatter and droplets. Whilst some surgical masks claim to have particulate filtration properties,

Table 6.3 Protection of the respiratory tract in dentistry

Source of particles	Size (diameter in microns)	Route of transmission	Protection
Splashing/ spraying	>100	Indirect contact with mucous membranes eyes, nose, mouth, skin of face	Eye protection Surgical mask
Droplets	5–100	Inhaled – penetrate the respiratory tract to above the alveolar level	Eye protection Surgical mask
Aerosols, e.g. from aerosol-generating procedures Droplet nuclei	<5	Inhaled – penetrate the respiratory system to the alveolar level	Eye protection Respirator mask Surgical mask offers limited protection – use risk assessment based on pathogen exposure*

* Respirator masks are recommended for aerosol-generating procedures involving body fluids, but their use in dentistry has been limited by the high unit cost.

they do not have the filtering efficiencies required for adequate respiratory protection against aerosols (see Table 6.3). Surgical masks are advocated for routine use in dentistry.

Masks come in various shapes (e.g. moulded and non-moulded) and method of attachment (e.g. ties and ear loops). They are disposable and intended for single use only. When worn correctly, the mask should cover the nose and mouth. If the mask is fitted with a metal nose band, this is contoured to the bridge of the nose. If the tapes are not sufficiently tight then the mask will leak around the sides and become ineffective. Nevertheless, most masks produce a relatively poor facial seal, and the air is not effectively filtered before inhalation into the lungs. Hence, masks provide minimal or partial protection of the wearer from respiratory pathogens spread by the aerosol route.

Good practice guide: how to use a surgical mask

- Masks are recommended for all dental procedures.
- Masks should be close fitting and cover the nose and mouth (Figure 6.2).
- Avoid touching the outer filtering surface of the mask, which may be contaminated.
- Only handle the ties/ear loops which are considered 'clean' and can be touched with bare hands.
- Masks are single-use items. They should be changed after every patient and not reused.
- Mask should be disposed of immediately after use as hazardous clinical infectious waste.
- Do not pull the surgical mask or respirator mask down to hang around the neck or wear on the elbow as this will lead to cross-contamination.

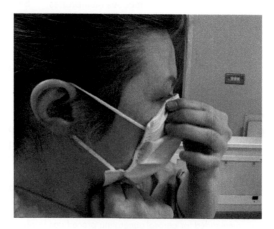

Figure 6.2 A mask being fitted to the facial contours.

- Hands should be cleaned after removing the mask in order to prevent contamination of your face and the surgery environment.

Respirator masks

> Respirator masks are used during the care of patients with respiratory infections transmitted by air-borne particles.

For a very small number of pathogens that are truly transmissible via the air-borne route, e.g. influenza virus, severe acute respiratory syndrome (SARS), *Mycobacterium tuberculosis*, an FFP3 respirator mask is recommended. An FFP3 respirator should be worn when carrying out aerosol-generating procedures, such as drilling on patients known or suspected to be infected with a micro-organism transmissible by the droplet and/or air-borne (aerosol) route. Compatible eye protection should always be worn. Importantly, it is worth noting that aerosol-generating procedures such as use of high-speed handpieces can generate an aerosol hazard from a microbe that ordinarily might only be transmissible via direct or indirect contact.

Respirator masks offer a higher degree of personal respiratory protection compared to a standard surgical face mask. They are designed to filter out air-borne particles smaller than 5 µm in the inspired air. These tiny particles are inhaled into the deepest part of the lung, the alveoli, where the microbes are then released and can cause infection. Only respirators with CE markings that conform to the latest European Standard EN149 should be worn. Respirator masks are sold with a range of filtering efficiencies. Outside the UK, respirator masks classified as FFP2 with 94% filtering efficiency (equivalent to American N95 masks) are recommended for use when treating patients with active tuberculosis (Figure 6.3). Masks with the highest level of filtering efficiency classified according to the European standard as FFP3 with 98% filtering efficiency are recommended by the UK Health and Safety Executive (HSE) for protection against infectious aerosols in healthcare (Figure 6.4). For example, such masks should be used when treating patients suffering from pandemic flu, measles, active MDR-tuberculosis, SARS, Ebola virus disease, varicella zoster and during aerosol-generating treatments on patients suffering from infections including, amongst others, influenza, norovirus, *Mycoplasma* pneumonia and rubella. It is envisaged that in most cases, only patients requiring emergency dental treatment are likely to attend when suffering from one of these conditions. Respirator masks must be fit tested and checked for facial seal by the wearer before use.

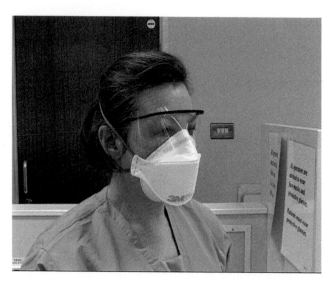

Figure 6.3 An FFP2 respirator mask worn with disposable safety goggles. These masks are recommended for use outside the UK.

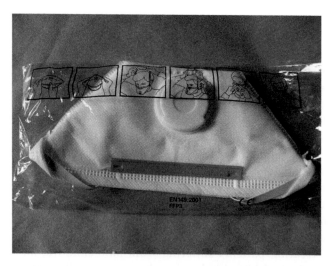

Figure 6.4 An FFP3 respirator mask. Note the valve to make breathing and wear more comfortable and the blue nose strip to enhance fit to the facial contour.

Good practice guide: fitting and wearing a respirator mask

- When fitted and worn correctly, respirators seal firmly to the face, thus reducing the risk of leakage.

- A facial seal check should be performed by the wearer of a respirator each time it is donned to minimize air leakage around the facepiece. These differ slightly with each product and are supplied by the manufacturer.
- Note that beards and stubble interfere with the fit and seal of the respirator.
- Avoid touching the outer surface of the respirator mask once it is fitted. Always clean hands after handling the mask.
- Dispose of as hazardous infectious clinical waste.

Respiratory hygiene

Surgical face masks are also advocated for respiratory hygiene. Lessons learnt during the SARS outbreak in 2003 demonstrated that infection was spread by undiagnosed patients coughing as they waited their turn for treatment in clinic waiting rooms. It is anticipated that cough etiquette protocols would become necessary in practice waiting areas during an outbreak of respiratory illness such as pandemic flu or for patients with active TB. In this situation, patients should be asked politely to wear a mask to prevent spread of infection from themselves to others. Alternatively, if patients are unwilling or unable to wear a mask, then they would be asked to cover the mouth/nose with a tissue when coughing and promptly dispose of used tissues and then clean their hands with alcohol-based hand rub. Ideally, patients should be seated more than 3 feet apart. Physical proximity of less than 3 feet from an infected person has been associated with increased droplet route transmission of bacteria such as *Neisseria meningitidis* and group A streptococcus.

PROTECTIVE EYEWEAR AND VISORS

The clinical dental team must protect their own eyes and those of the patient against respiratory secretions, splatter, aerosols and foreign bodies such as amalgam fragments. Eye protection is always required during potentially infectious aerosol-generating procedures. Spectacles and contact lenses are not considered adequate eye protection. Ideally, eye protection (goggles or visor/face shields) should be comfortable and allow for sufficient peripheral vision and secure fit, and offer protection from splashes, sprays and respiratory droplets from multiple angles. Many styles of goggles fit adequately over spectacles with minimal gaps or a visor can be worn (Figure 6.5). A visor can be worn over loupes and protect the eyepieces from contamination. While effective as eye protection, goggles do not provide splash or spray protection to other parts of the face. Use of goggles was shown to protect the wearer from occupational infection with respiratory syncytial virus (RSV) which is spread by respiratory

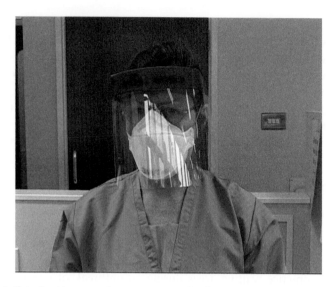

Figure 6.5 If the healthcare worker wears spectacles then a visor or goggles should be worn over the mask. *Note*: A visor does not provide protection from respiratory aerosols, so a mask is worn under it.

droplets. Whether this was due to preventing hand–eye contact or respiratory droplet–eye contact has not been determined. Careful fitting of eyewear and masks before patient contact avoids the need to make further adjustments to the PPE during treatment. Whenever possible, avoid touching your mouth, nose, eyes or face with contaminated hands or gloves.

Goggles provide suitable protection for the eyes when splashing is likely, whilst face shields are best worn where there is a risk of blood or body fluid splattering or spraying of potentially infectious material as they provide full-face protection. Eye protection should ideally be disposable but if this is not possible then it should be decontaminated following use.

Good practice guide: goggles and face shields

- Goggles with side protection or face shields should be worn during all types of dental treatment or when manually cleaning instruments.
- Single-use disposable goggles and visors are preferred but reusable goggles and visors should be decontaminated according to the manufacturer's instructions for cleaning the surface with disinfectant, e.g. alcohol-based surface disinfectant wipe.
- Goggles should not impair the operator's vision as this could result in compromised patient care. If they become scratched or cloudy following multiple use, they should be replaced.
- In the event of contamination of the eyes with blood or other body fluids or chemicals, first remove contact lens (if worn) and then rinse the eye with

copious amounts of eye wash or cold water. If the source patient is a carrier of a blood-borne virus then follow the advice for managing a sharps/splash incident outlined in Chapter 4.

The World Health Organization (WHO) recommends that PPE should be donned and removed in the following order to minimize environmental and self-contamination.

Good practice guide: donning protective equipment

- Perform hand hygiene
- Plastic apron (or fluid-repellent gown)
- Surgical mask (or respirator mask)
- Protective eyewear
- Gloves

Good practice guide: removing protective equipment

- Gloves
- Plastic apron or gown
- Protective eyewear
- Mask or respirator mask
- Perform hand hygiene

Gloves are removed first as they are contaminated on their outer surface with the patient's secretions and this manoeuvre then prevents you from touching and potentially infecting your own skin, eyes or mouth whilst removing the other contaminated items of PPE. See Figure 6.6 for glove removal technique. Gloves should be removed immediately after completing treatment even if other items of PPE are not removed to prevent contamination of inanimate surfaces in the surgery environment. Masks are removed by handling the ties or earpieces only. Dispose of single-use PPE and RPE immediately into hazardous infectious clinical waste sacks. Reuseable items should be decontaminated.

PROTECTION DURING CARDIOPULMONARY RESUSCITATION

Mouthpieces, pocket resuscitation masks with one-way valves and other ventilation devices provide a safe alternative to mouth-to-mouth resuscitation, preventing exposure of the caregiver's nose and mouth to oral and respiratory fluids during the procedure

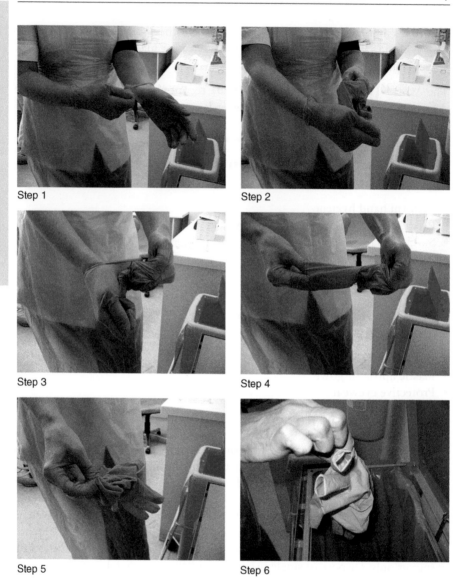

Step 1

Step 2

Step 3

Step 4

Step 5

Step 6

Figure 6.6 Stages of aseptic glove removal to prevent contamination of the wearer's hands and the environment.

TUNICS AND UNIFORMS

Prevent tunics and uniforms becoming a source of infection.

Uniform styles

After a day working in the dental surgery, tunic, trousers and uniform will have become progressively contaminated with microbes from several sources, including the wearer's skin organisms, the patient's pathogens and environmental micro-organisms. In hospital wards, multidrug-resistant bacteria (MRSA), *Clostridium difficile* and vancomycin-resistant enterococci have been transmitted from patient to patient via contaminated uniforms, but transmission via this route appears to be uncommon.

In dentistry, splatter generated during the use of rotary equipment falls mainly on the operator's face, chest, hands and wrists. Neck ties have been implicated in transmission of MRSA. Ties (except for bow ties) and dangling necklaces should not be worn when treating patients, or if worn should be concealed under the tunic and uniform. High-necked tunics and uniforms that cover the upper chest area are therefore advised.

Working bare below the elbow

The current mantra is for working 'bare below the elbows', i.e. short sleeves, with no watches or jewellery in order to facilitate effective hand hygiene (Figure 6.7). Long sleeves become wet during hand washing and wet fabric promotes the survival and growth of bacteria. Long sleeves and dangling cuffs are also vulnerable to direct contamination by splatter generated by handpieces and respiratory droplets expelled from the patient's mouth. Remember, however, when wearing short-sleeved uniforms that the wrists and forearms will be covered with microbes after dental treatment and will need to be cleaned thoroughly.

Good practice guide: wearing and cleaning of workwear

- Uniforms should be changed daily or more frequently if visibly soiled with body fluids or obvious stains such as ink from leaking biros, oil stains, etc.
- Protective clothing should not be worn in designated eating and rest areas within the practice. Remove protective clothing when eating and drinking.
- Tunics and uniforms should be removed before leaving the practice and placed in an impermeable bag.
- Do not 'greet' friends and family with pathogens picked up in the surgery.
- When purchasing uniforms, it makes sense to choose fabrics and colours that can tolerate washing at the higher temperatures required to kill microbes.

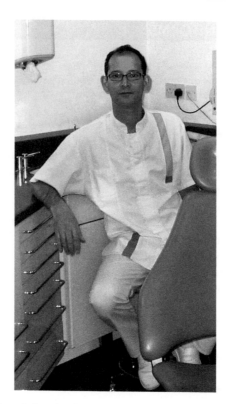

Figure 6.7 Working bare below the elbow. The dentist is wearing a short-sleeved, high-neckline tunic and no watch is worn.

- Tunics/uniforms should be washed separately from the household wash in a washing machine set on a hot wash (preferably 60 °C or above for 10 minutes), which will destroy many bacteria except heat-resistant spore formers. A 40 °C wash temperature is acceptable but removal of microbes is then reliant on the dilution effect of the rinse water and detergent action, which is less reliable.
- Detergents release microbes and dirt from the fabric, which are then removed in the rinse water. Avoid overloading the machine as this will reduce the dilution effect of rinsing.
- Iron the uniform, as the heat generated by ironing will help to destroy any bacteria remaining on the clothes. Ironing without prior washing reduces microbial counts by approximately 10^7 cfu/mL but is not sufficient on its own.
- If dental staff wear their own clothes in the dental practice then similar hygiene measures should be employed.

Tunic and uniforms are not PPE.

Tunics and uniforms are not considered PPE as they are usually made of materials such as polycottons that are permeable to micro-organisms and body fluids. Uniforms are not a substitute for barrier protection with PPE (plastic aprons or fluid-repellent gowns). Rather, uniforms reflect the practice's corporate image and fulfil the patient's expectation of how members of the dental team, including trainees and students, should be dressed.

Staff should be permitted to dress in accordance with their religious and cultural practices, as long as this does not interfere with good infection control practice. In the dental surgery whilst performing hand and wrist hygiene and during patient treatment, the uniform or workwear sleeves should be pushed up over the elbow and secured in place. A disposable long-sleeved gown or disposable over-sleeve can be worn to cover the bare forearm during patient treatment (Figure 6.8). The cuff of the glove should cover the cuff of the disposable 'sleeve'. Remember, over-sleeves are single-use items. They must be changed between patients and disposed of as infectious clinical waste. However, the uniform dress code should allow for covering of the forearm at other times with long sleeves.

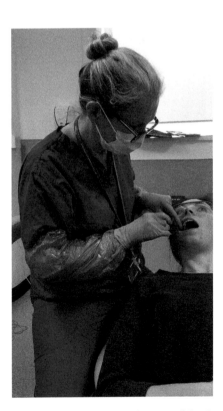

Figure 6.8 A disposable over-sleeve worn to cover the arms of the dentist during treatment.

PERSONAL PROTECTION FOR PREVENTION OF CROSS-INFECTION

PROTECTIVE BARRIERS – PLASTIC APRONS AND SURGICAL GOWNS

Plastic aprons

> Protect yourself from splatter with a disposable plastic apron.

National and international recommendations on standard precautions state that healthcare workers should wear disposable plastic aprons to protect the front of their uniform/clothing from microbial contamination arising from close contact with patients, materials and contaminated equipment or splatter. They are considered suitable for general clinical use, manual instrument cleaning or mopping up body fluid spills. If extensive exposure to blood or body fluids is expected then fluid-repellent disposable gowns are appropriate (Figure 6.9).

Plastic aprons are classified as single-use items and should be changed between patients or each procedure and then discarded as hazardous clinical waste. They are prone to develop static electric charge in use, which attracts increased numbers of bacteria onto the apron (Figure 6.10). So, care must be

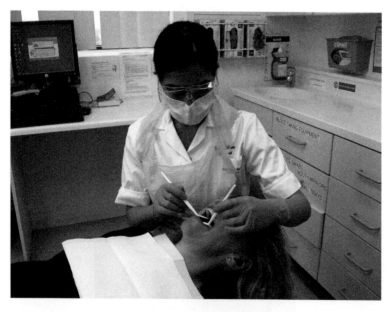

Figure 6.9 Dentist wearing a disposable single-use plastic apron, which is designed to protect the wearer from splatter falling on the chest and waist area of the body, when working in the seated position.

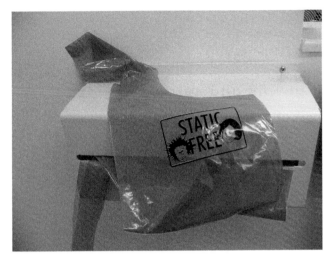

Figure 6.10 Antistatic disposable aprons in a wall-mounted dispenser.

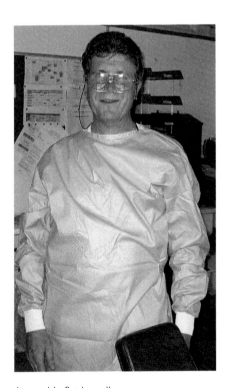

Figure 6.11 Single-use disposable fluid-repellent gown.

taken to avoid touching the outer surface of the apron during wear or disposal; however, antistatic versions are available. Stocks of plastic aprons should be stored in a clean, dust-free place.

Surgical gowns and surgical drapes

If there is a risk of splashing with blood or body fluids onto skin or clothing such as during minor oral surgery, periodontal or implant surgery then disposable, long-sleeved fluid-repellent surgical gowns are advised (Figure 6.11). Gowns are usually the first piece of PPE to be donned after hand hygiene has been performed. Gowns should have long sleeves with tight-fitting cuffs. Gloves are worn over the cuff of the sleeve, which protects the wrists from contamination and helps to prevent wetting of the cuff. When removing the gown, the outer, 'contaminated' side of the gown is folded inwards and rolled into a bundle, and then discarded into a hazardous waste receptacle. Make every effort to avoid touching the outer contaminated surface of the gown.

REFERENCES AND WEBSITES

Coia JE, Ritchie L, Adisesh A *et al.* for the Healthcare Infection Society Working Group on Respiratory and Facial Protection (2013) Guidance on the use of respiratory and facial protection equipment. *Journal of Hospital Infection*, **85**, 170–182.

Loveday HP, Wilson JA, Pratta RJ *et al.* (2014) Epic3: national evidence-based guidelines for preventing healthcare-associated infections in NHS hospitals in England. *Journal of Hospital Infection*, **86**(Suppl. 1), S1–S70.

Seto WH, Tsang D, Yung RWH *et al.* (2003) Effectiveness of precautions against droplets and contact in prevention of nosocomial transmission of severe acute respiratory syndrome (SARS). *Lancet*, **361**, 1519–1520.

Chapter 7

Sterilization and disinfection of dental instruments

DECONTAMINATION CYCLE

Decontamination is performed for two important reasons.

- To make a reusable device safe for staff to handle.
- To minimize (i.e. disinfect) or eliminate the risk of transmission of infection from one patient to another (i.e. sterilization).

The ultimate goal is to produce a sterile instrument that is completely free of all micro-organisms. Sterilization is not sufficient on its own to achieve this aim. Instruments cannot be sterilized unless they are first cleaned because debris (cement, blood, lubricant oil, etc.) adhering to the surface of an instrument can inhibit or interfere with the sterilization process. Therefore, decontamination is an incremental process with each stage (Figure 7.1) contributing to the killing and removal of micro-organisms.

Definitions:

- *cleaning*: physical removal (including prions) but not necessarily killing of microbes
- *disinfection*: reduction of the microbial load to a level that makes the disinfected object safe to handle
- *sterilization*: killing and removal of all micro-organisms including bacterial spores.

Many vegetative (non-spore-forming) bacteria are killed at temperatures above 60–65 °C. Spore-forming bacteria and *Mycobacteria* spp. have protective cell walls that make them relatively resistant to thermal killing. To destroy these organisms, the higher temperatures generated during steam sterilization under

Basic Guide to Infection Prevention and Control in Dentistry, Second Edition.
Caroline L. Pankhurst.
© 2017 John Wiley & Sons Ltd. Published 2017 by John Wiley & Sons Ltd.
Companion website: www.wiley.com/go/pankhurst/infection-prevention

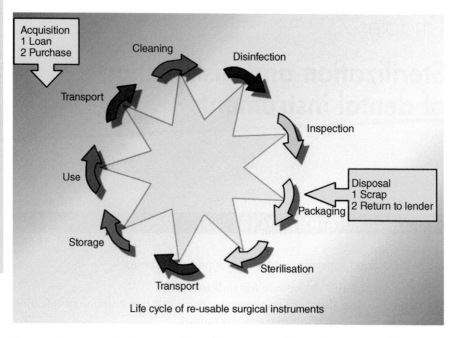

Figure 7.1 Decontamination cycle of reusable instruments. Source: Courtesy of Paul Morris.

pressure are necessary. Unfortunately, prion proteins such vCJD or CJD are highly resistant to thermal killing, and removal and destruction of prions are reliant for the most part on effective cleaning and disinfection.

Complete removal of the bacterial cell is necessary as endotoxin derived from the cell wall of dead Gram-negative bacteria, though not infectious, can trigger an inflammatory reaction. In addition, a decontaminated instrument whether disinfected or sterilized should be free from:

- residues of previous clinical treatment, e.g. cement, microbes, blood and human tissue
- residues from the decontamination process, e.g. detergents, disinfectants and limescale
- contamination during storage by dust, dirt and environmental microbial contamination.

WHY HAS CLEANING BECOME SO IMPORTANT?

Prion proteins are more resistant to sterilization.

Cleaning has always been an important component of the decontamination process, but has increased in significance as a result of the emergence of transmissible prion disease (variant Creutzfeldt–Jakob disease – vCJD), which first appeared in humans in the mid-1990s (see Chapter 2). Prion diseases are rare, fatal, neurodegenerative disorders. CJD occurs naturally in human populations as a sporadic or familial condition at a rate of approximately 1.5 cases per million population per annum. Iatrogenic cases are associated with transmission from contaminated instruments or grafts during neurosurgical procedures, and in the past from human-derived growth hormone. Prions, unlike other pathogens, contain no DNA or RNA but are composed of a protein with an abnormal conformation. Proteins are considerably more resistant to thermal denaturation than DNA or RNA. Sterilization reduces infectivity (i.e. deactivation of prion agents) only by 100- to 1000-fold. There is evidence that prions are modified by adsorption onto a metal surface, making them more resistant to decontamination.

Normally, to initiate an infection from a surgical instrument, the micro-organism requires a method of transmission to transfer it from the surface of the instrument into the patient's bloodstream or tissues and this is usually achieved through the percutaneous route or by direct contact. This sequence of events is unnecessary for transmission of prion disease, as infection can be initiated even when the agent remains adherent to the instrument. Once present on an instrument, the prion can continue to 'infect' patients until it is physically removed.

Prion proteins are destroyed by strong alkalis, but such compounds can damage instruments, making them unsuitable for routine use. A number of alternative solutions have been developed to deactivate prion proteins, including radiofrequency-generated gas plasma machines and prion-degrading enzyme disinfectants. However, routine decontamination focuses on effective cleaning protocols to physically remove all proteins, including prions.

Previously, the benchmark standard for cleaning was 'reduction of bacterial load', but now it has been raised to the 'removal of prion proteins'. On a practical level, this change is translated into the replacement of manual cleaning by automated cleaning, preferably with a thermal washer disinfector. However dedicated the person cleaning the dental instruments, all manual procedures are subject to operator variation as a result of time constraints or tiredness. Automated cleaning has the major advantage of being reproducible and open to validation. Validation is defined as the means by which an entire process is documented, tested and able to be repeated.

LEGAL REQUIREMENTS AND TECHNICAL STANDARDS FOR DECONTAMINATION

Complying with the law

Sterilizers and thermal washer disinfectors are classified under Medical Devices Regulations (MDR) 2002 in the UK and by European Union law as medical devices. Both the equipment and the site where decontamination takes place are required to operate according to the MDR. Medical devices manufactured and marketed within the UK and throughout the EU are subject to specific regulation and must carry a CE marking. This denotes compliance with a range of essential test requirements covering the safety and performance of the medical device. Decontaminated instruments and equipment must conform to two fundamental principles in order to be compliant with the MDR.

- Be clean and sterile at the end of the decontamination process.
- Be maintained in a clinically satisfactory condition up to the point of use.

The basic standards that are applicable for the management and operation of the decontamination process in the UK are summarized in Box 7.1.

Reusable dental instruments and equipment are decontaminated to one of the following three levels:

Box 7.1   Basic principles for the management of decontamination in a dental practice

- Nominate a decontamination lead person with responsibility for establishment and implementation of a standardized decontamination process in the practice, with line management responsibility to the registered provider/manager (practice owner).

- Undertake sterilization in dedicated facilities outside the patient treatment room and store sterile instruments in a dedicated clean area. Facilities need to be fit for purpose, well organized and maintained.

- Restrict manual cleaning to those items incompatible with automated processes. Clean compatible instruments using an automated process, e.g. thermal washer disinfector.

- Decontamination equipment must be fit for purpose. Fully validate equipment before use to ensure that it is functioning correctly.

- Perform maintenance, service and daily, weekly and annual periodic testing in accordance with current national recommendations.

- Record and retain all validation and periodic testing documentation to demonstrate that each part of the process has been effective in preparation for external audit or inspections for a minimum of two years.

- Operate a documented training scheme and keep individual training records for all personnel involved in decontamination. Staff need to know their specific roles and be fully trained to carry out their duties effectively.

- Undertake regular audit* and review to monitor whether processes are up to date, are being followed and to implement any changes required. Completed audits and action plans should be stored and be available for inspection as part of the practice's risk management system.

Source: Compiled from HTM 01-05 and Scottish Dental Clinical Effectiveness Programme.

* Biannual in HTM 01-05.

Table 7.1 Risk assessment for decontamination of instruments and equipment

Risk	Application	Recommendation
High (critical)	Penetrates soft tissue, contacts bone or enters a normally sterile body tissue or bloodstream or items used in close contact with a break in the skin or mucous membrane	Sterile (at point of use) or commercial sterile single-use instruments
Medium (semi-critical)	In contact with non-intact skin, mucous membranes or body fluid	Sterilized
Low (non-critical)	In contact with intact skin or does not come in contact with the patient	Cleaning

- sterile (at point of use)
- sterilized (i.e. having been through the sterilization process)
- clean (i.e. free of visible contamination).

The choice is made based on a risk assessment of the degree of instrument penetration, contact or non-contact with skin, mucous membranes, sterile body cavities or bloodstream (Table 7.1).

Technical standards for decontamination

There are agreed British/European technical standards for the manufacture and operation of sterilizers and washer disinfectors, e.g. British/European standards, BS EN ISO 15883 (washer disinfectors) and BS EN ISO 13060 (bench-top sterilizers). These BS/EN technical standards are incorporated into the clinical decontamination technical guidance published nationally to help dental practices achieve a safe and effective standard of instrument decontamination (e.g. HTM 01-05, and in Scotland SHTM 2010 and SDCEP Decontamination into practice). In addition, these national guidelines act as benchmarks for the purposes of registration, audit and external inspection of dental practices in the UK (see Box 7.1). Practice owners/registered providers/ managers are obliged to be familiar with the content of these documents, to appoint an infection control and decontamination lead, to undertake regular decontamination audits and to train their staff accordingly. Completed audits and subsequent action plans provide evidence for practice inspectors that the dental practice has a valid quality assurance and risk management system in place for decontamination.

However, the underlying scientific principles on which these regulations and guidelines are based are universal, and are applicable wherever the reader is practising dentistry and decontaminating dental instruments and equipment. The fine detail in interpreting these basic principles may vary from country to country and examples can be viewed by clicking on the hyperlinks in the companion website and in the reference list at the end of the chapter.

WHERE SHOULD INSTRUMENT DECONTAMINATION TAKE PLACE?

Currently, sterilization of equipment for use in dentistry takes place within the dental practice, but this is not the only option available.

1. Outsource decontamination to an accredited sterile services department (SSD).
2. Use CE-marked single-use medical devices.
3. Undertake local decontamination to national standards (e.g. HTM 01-05 or equivalent).
4. Combination of 1–3.

For example, option 1 is considered the preferred method by many specialists in decontamination but logistical considerations limit its use to dental instrument decontamination undertaken in dental hospitals, the acute sector and health board clinics. Most, but not all, dental practices will probably opt for option 4, i.e. to continue local decontamination combined with selective use of disposable instruments. As we have seen in the previous section, this puts the onus on the dental practice to comply with the national standards, which are outlined in brief in Box 7.1. Note that validation of the decontamination cycle is considered as important as the design of the decontamination room and the type of equipment used within it. The next part of this chapter will outline how these goals can be achieved.

DESIGN OF DEDICATED DECONTAMINATION UNITS

Best practice guidelines in the UK for instrument decontamination include:

- a dedicated decontamination room
- a separate sterile instrument storage area
- use of a validated washer disinfector to replace manual cleaning wherever possible.

Ideally, a dental surgery (treatment room) would be used exclusively for clinical treatment and should not be used for any part of the decontamination cycle. Why is this? Primarily, the aim is to ensure both the patient's safety and quality assurance of the sterilization process. Each step of the decontamination process aims to reduce the microbial load on the instruments. Therefore, it is crucial that clean and dirty instruments are segregated and instruments are not recontaminated after cleaning or sterilization by direct contact with contaminated surfaces, splashes or aerosols generated during patient treatment. Conversely, moving instrument decontamination out of the treatment area protects the patient from contaminated aerosols generated during cleaning instruments used on previous patients.

Furthermore, a sterilizer is a pressurized item of equipment, and the pressure that builds up behind the door of the sterilizer is equivalent to 750 kg or three-quarters of a ton. If the door fails, which occasionally happens, then the sterilizer effectively becomes a bomb, capable of causing considerable damage to anything in its path. If the sterilizer is housed on the work surface in a small surgery, the patient or members of the dental team could be seriously hurt during such an incident.

Therefore, all these safety requirements can be met by undertaking the decontamination cycle within a dedicated decontamination facility. Segregation between those instruments awaiting decontamination and disinfected and sterile instruments can be achieved in several ways.

- A single-room decontamination facility (Figure 7.2) with a one-way flow of instruments and pattern of working from dirty to clean. The thermal washer disinfector is placed at the junction between the dirty and clean areas (see Figure 7.3). To prevent aerosol cross-contamination, the room is ventilated by use of a controlled air flow in the direction opposite to that of the instrument

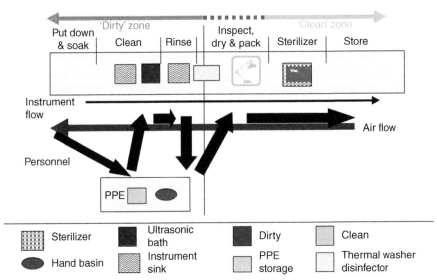

Figure 7.2 Basic design for a one-room decontamination facility. A second hand basin in the clean zone is optional.

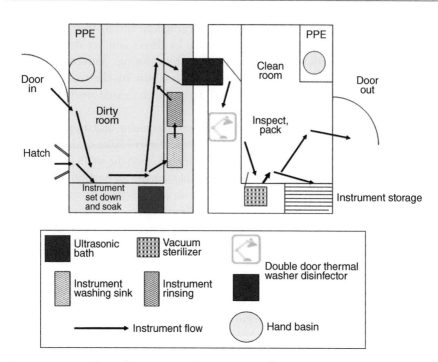

Figure 7.3 Basic design for a two-room decontamination facility.

flow, i.e. from clean to dirty. A through-the-wall or window fan-based ventilation and extraction system is recommended. This is not foolproof as air flows can be disrupted by opening the doors or windows or by movement of personnel in the room. Do not use portable fans in the decontamination area as they can circulate contamination around the room and destroy the clean-to-dirty air flow. Figure 7.2 shows movement patterns of personnel within the room to maintain the zoning. It requires a high level of staff discipline and training to achieve this work flow pattern and therefore is more prone to human error than in a two-room facility.

- A two-room decontamination facility with one room for decontamination of dirty instruments and the second room for sterilization, packaging and storage of cleaned instruments is illustrated in Figure 7.3. A double-door washer disinfector is inserted in the wall/barrier between the dirty and clean rooms (Figure 7.4). The illustrated design shows how controlled access to the rooms can be achieved via the addition of a hand-through hatch (for the delivery of dirty sets of instruments and equipment); an alternative method is shown in Figure 7.5. A two-room design is the preferred option as cross-contamination is unlikely to occur. It most closely mimics the tried-and-tested layout used in hospital sterile services departments. However, this design is most effective when there is a dedicated member of staff working in the decontamination suite.

(a)

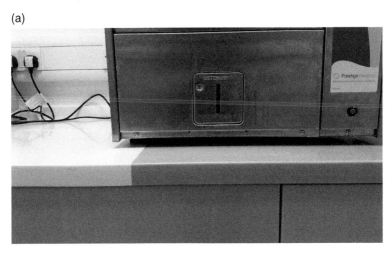

(b)

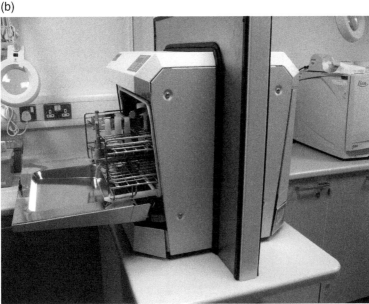

Figure 7.4 Demonstration of two different methods to clearly demarcate the clean and the dirty zones in a one-room decontamination facility. (a) Different colour benchtop (white and grey) to demarcate clean and dirty zones. The junction between the zones is at the thermal washer disinfector. (b) Simple glass divider at the junction of the clean and dirty areas, which houses a two-door thermal washer disinfector. As a method to prevent cross-contamination, when one door is open the other is automatically locked shut.

In both options, instruments are transported to and from the treatment room in rigid, leak-proof containers with secure lids (Figure 7.6). Designate one clearly labelled container for the transport of clean instruments and a second for the transport of dirty instruments. Containers should be cleaned and disinfected

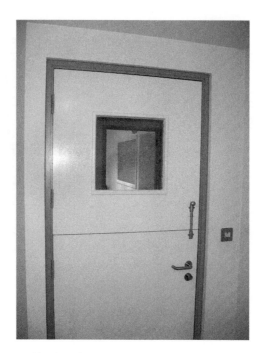

Figure 7.5 Two-part stable door for controlled access. The top part of the door can be opened and used as a pass-through instrument hatch.

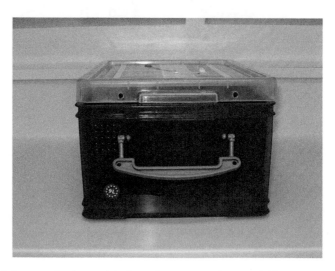

Figure 7.6 An example of a rigid, leak-proof container with secure lid for instrument transportation to the decontamination suite from the dental surgery.

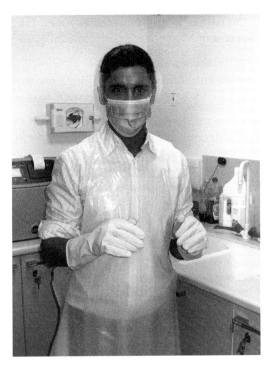

Figure 7.7 Demonstrating the personal protective equipment worn for instrument cleaning, including visor (or goggles), mask, plastic apron and heavy-duty gloves.

between each use, preferably by disinfection in a thermal washer disinfector. Avoid the use of bleach or hypochlorite solution because any residues might damage the instruments. Staff should clean their hands and put on personal protective equipment (PPE) on entering the decontamination facility and remove PPE and clean hands on exiting (see Chapters 5 and 6) (Figure 7.7). In addition, they should clean their hands and change their PPE when shifting from working in the dirty zone to the clean zone, in order to prevent cross-contamination (see Figure 7.2 and Box 7.2).

Temporal separation

The illustrated designs are for 'ideal' decontamination facilities and the interpretation of the Medical Devices Directive is not uniform across the EU or even the UK. But the fundamental principle of segregating dirty and clean procedures applies even when the decontamination is performed in the treatment room, as patient safety is paramount. In the latter situation, a degree of separation can be achieved by introducing some simple measures. Temporal separation (separating activities in time) can be used to conduct different activities in the same space. Patient safety can be enhanced by not decontaminating instruments while the patient is in the treatment room. The following decontamination procedures should not take place while the patient is present:

- manual instrument washing and rinsing
- opening of decontamination equipment, e.g. ultrasonic bath, thermal washer disinfector or sterilizer. Only operate the ultrasonic bath with the lid closed.

Most surgeries have two sinks, one for the nurse and the other for the dentist, and one of these can be designated as the dedicated sink for instrument cleaning

---

Box 7.2   Basic design requirements

Decontamination rooms should contain the following features
- An uncluttered, single run of sealed, impermeable, easily cleaned worktop
- A wash hand basin and storage for personal protective equipment (PPE) in the dirty zone. If space allows, place a second wash hand basin and storage for PPE in the clean zone (optional but include in the design of a two-room suite)
- An entry door into the dirty zone, an exit door out of the clean zone (a second door is optional)

Dirty room/zone (instrument soaking, cleaning and disinfection)
- A setdown area to receive dirty instruments and for precleaning soaking of instruments
- A deep instrument washing sink with detergent dispenser and a set-down area for washed instruments. Alternatively, a double sink unit consisting of two bowls, one for washing and one for rinsing with a common supply tap
- Ultrasonic bath (an optional item – can be placed before the washing sink or between the two sinks to facilitate rinsing of instruments cleaned in the ultrasonic bath)
- An instrument rinsing sink and set-down area for rinsed instruments
- Thermal washer disinfector

Clean room/zone (inspection, sterilization and storage)
- A setting-down area with task lighting and magnifier for inspection of all instruments and, if appropriate, a dental handpiece lubricator
- An area for wrapping instruments (only if a vacuum sterilizer installed) (Figure 7.8)
- A steam sterilizer(s) (N, B or S type)
- A clean, well-lit area for unloading the sterilizer (and for instrument packing, if instruments are sterilized in non-vacuum sterilizer)
- A clean, dry, enclosed instrument storage area which is away from direct sunlight, with orderly storage for stock control and sufficient access to permit stock rotation. Avoid the use of open shelving and do not store instruments on the floor
- Water for steam generation can be purchased or produced on site using a still to make distilled water or a reverse osmosis machine. Space has to be allowed for this equipment and for storing one day's supply of water

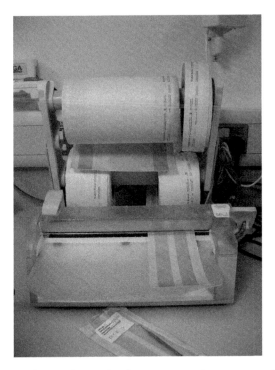

Figure 7.8 Heat sealing machine in the clean zone to seal instrument packs either before or after sterilization. The machine is fitted with rolls of packaging of different sizes suitable for use with a range of trays sizes or for packing single instruments.

STERILIZATION AND DISINFECTION OF DENTAL INSTRUMENTS

and rinsing. Manual washing requires separate washing and rinsing sinks/ bowls to prevent recontamination of the cleaned instruments. Best practice recommends the use of two separate instrument sinks. If space is at a premium then the use of a removable plastic or metal bowl for rinsing is permitted as an interim measure. Recontamination of instruments can be reduced by thorough surface disinfection of the worktops between the dirty and clean stages of decontamination. Adequate ventilation and exhaust air extraction in the region of 10–12 air changes per hour or higher in the treatment room will help to reduce air contamination to a low level.

PURCHASING OF DENTAL EQUIPMENT

Dental devices marketed in the EU carry a CE mark, which indicates that the equipment is 'fit for the intended purpose'. Manufacturers of medical/dental devices must by law provide decontamination instruction methods for cleaning, disinfection and sterilization and state any limit to the number of times an item can be sterilized. Before you purchase a new item, it is prudent to check the manufacturer's decontamination instructions to ensure that the instruments can be decontaminated with the facilities that you have available in the practice or dental school. When choosing new instruments, it is good practice to purchase instruments that can be cleaned using an automated method. Alternatively, you could consider replacing difficult-to-clean instruments with single-use instruments.

CLEANING OF DENTAL INSTRUMENTS

Automated versus manual cleaning

Instruments can be cleaned manually or by machine using an ultrasonic bath and/or a thermal washer disinfector. According to best practice, manual cleaning of instruments should be restricted to those items incompatible with automated washing. Studies have demonstrated that washer disinfectors are more efficient at reducing the bacterial load during presterilization cleaning than either ultrasonic cleaning or manual cleaning of dental instruments. Staff safety is enhanced as instruments do not need to be scrubbed, so there is less exposure to pathogenic micro-organisms, sharps injuries or noxious chemicals. Overall productivity is increased in the dental practice as more time becomes available for clinical activities. There are, however, some disadvantages to thermal disinfectors. Manual cleaning is faster than using a thermal washer disinfector. The average downtime for instruments cleaned and dried in a thermal washer disinfector and sterilized in a vacuum sterilizer is approximately two hours, necessitating the purchase of additional instruments if the same numbers of patients are to be seen.

Preventing corrosion of instruments

Proteins in blood and saliva left on the instrument after treatment are absorbed and then fixed onto the surface of the instrument. Fixation is a chemical process that takes about 30 minutes at room temperature, but is faster at higher temperatures. Eventually, blood and saline will corrode stainless steel instruments, leading to pitting and rusting of the surface. Damaged and pitted instruments are more difficult to clean effectively and rust or corrosion reduces the life of the instrument. Ideally, instruments should be cleaned as soon as possible after use, i.e. within 10 minutes. If it is not practical to clean the instruments immediately then soak them in a non-ionic or enzymatic detergent solution, precleaning foam/gel or store in a humid environment. Do avoid soaking in plain water for long periods as this can lead to instrument corrosion and rusting and can enhance prion affinity for the instrument surface.

Manual cleaning of instruments

> Manual cleaning carries an inoculation injury and inhalation risk.

Manual cleaning as a process cannot be directly validated so according to best practice quality standards cannot be used as the sole method of cleaning. It is reserved only for instruments or equipment which according to the manufacturer cannot be cleaned by an automated process or when the washer disinfector is temporarily unavailable. In England, it is still permitted as the sole cleaning method as best practice was not mandatory at the time of writing this chapter.

Manual cleaning lowers the bacterial load on a used instrument by log 10^{3-4}, i.e. by 1000 to 10000-fold. Cleaning dental instruments should not be treated in the same way as washing up a coffee cup at home! Personnel undertaking instrument decontamination should be trained in manual cleaning using a written method, even when the practice routinely employs automated methods. A back-up cleaning protocol is invaluable for times when the thermal disinfector is undergoing maintenance and validation or if an instrument fails to be cleaned satisfactorily and requires additional cleaning.

Passive layer and choice of cleaning agents

In dentistry, we work with high-quality stainless steel instruments that are fabricated from chromium-rich steel, which forms a protective passive layer that allows the instrument to withstand the wear and tear of clinical use. If damaged, the passive layer has the capability to self-heal in the presence of air but this property is destroyed by the action of bleach or abrasive metal brushes. Therefore, only use CE marked detergents and disinfectants, which are marketed specifically for instrument decontamination. They are designed not to damage the passive surface layer and are tested for their antimicrobial activity and performance. Disinfectant and detergents will perform most effectively at the manufacturer's recommended concentrations. For manual or automated cleaning of instruments, the published guidelines recommend the use of a non-foaming detergent, with a pH 5–9, dispensed in a measured dose to be added to a measured volume of water at temperature below 45 °C. Lukewarm water prevents precipitation of proteins and fixation of blood and saliva to the instrument surface, making the nurse's job easier. Always remember to take great care when handling sharp instruments, especially as many hand instruments are sharp at both ends (see Chapter 4).

Personal protective clothing

Before cleaning the instruments, the staff member should put on the following protective clothing.

- Disposable plastic apron
- Face shield or eyewear
- Face mask
- Heavy-duty household gloves (surgical gloves should not be worn). When moving from working in a designated dirty area to a clean area, change gloves and plastic apron and clean hands

Good practice guide: manual instruments cleaning

- Use dedicated deep sinks (separate washing and rinsing sinks).
- Use a non-foaming detergent (do *not* use washing-up liquid, which leaves a residue and the surface foam impedes visibility of sharp instruments).
- Use a thermometer to measure the water temperature or use a temperature-sensitive detergent (water hotter than 45 °C will coagulate proteins and inhibit their removal).
- Measure the volume of water and detergent to give the concentration specified by the manufacturer. A line can be drawn on the sink to indicate the correct depth for the water. Add the detergent to the water, as this produces fewer bubbles.
- Instruments should be fully immersed and cleaned below the waterline to reduce aerosol formation. Instruments should not be held directly under a running tap, as this is likely to generate splashes and aerosols.
- Use a long-handled nylon brush, *not* abrasive pads or wire brushes. Cleaning equipment (e.g. plastic bristle brushes) should be cleaned and sterilized (or alternatively use disposables) and stored dry between use. Brushes should not be stored in disinfectant solutions. Replace regularly.
- Disassemble multipart instruments; pay special attention to crevices and joints.
- Rinse instruments in a separate rinsing sink. Care should be taken to avoid splashing and generating aerosols. Keep instruments submerged when rinsing.
- Dry instruments with non-linting disposable paper towel.
- Visually inspect instruments using an illuminated magnifier for damage, residual debris or blood and repeat cleaning stage if necessary (Figure 7.9). Remove and discard instruments with rust spots.
- Both sinks must be drained off and the sinks and work surfaces must be cleaned after use.
- Instruments should be sterilized as soon as possible after cleaning to avoid corrosion and/or microbial regrowth.
- New dental instruments must be cleaned and sterilized before they are used for the first time unless they are supplied as sterile by the manufacturer.

(a)

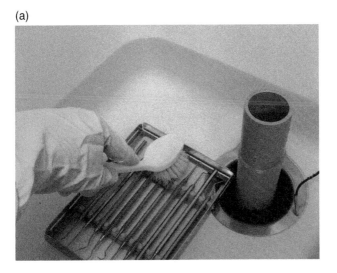

(b)

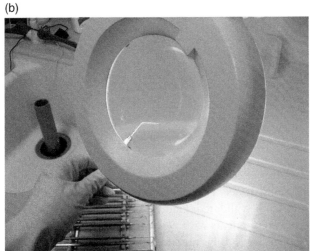

Figure 7.9 Manual cleaning of instruments. (a) Keep instruments immersed during cleaning. Note the use of a standpipe plug, which acts as an overflow as instrument washing sinks like hand basins are constructed without overflows. (b) Inspecting an instrument for residual debris or rust spots using an illuminated magnifier. Dispose of rusted instruments.

DISINFECTION OF DENTAL HANDPIECES

Automated methods

Best practice is to use an automated method to clean and disinfect dental handpieces with the aid of a thermal washer disinfector or an automated handpiece cleaner/sterilizer such as DAC machine. Where the manufacturer does not

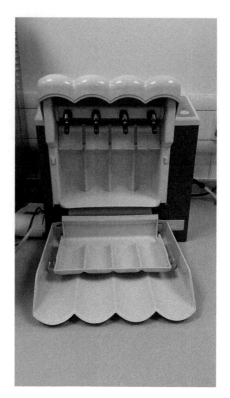

Figure 7.10 Dental handpiece cleaning and lubricating machine, which cleans up to four handpieces.

recommend disinfection with a thermal washer disinfector then consider using a handpiece-cleaning device. These devices only clean and lubricate, they do not disinfect and cannot be validated (Figure 7.10). They use a pressurized system to clean the internal components with detergent and then lubricate the handpieces with oil. Finally, the excess oil is purged, which reduces the amount of carryover of oil into the sterilizer, and the interior is dried with compressed air.

Most modern contralateral, straight and turbine handpieces are thermal washer disinfector tolerant and carry the washer disinfector safe symbol (Figure 7.11). Thermal washer disinfectors are fitted with plug-in connectors for dental handpieces that ensure that the internal lumens are disinfected. If recommended by the manufacturer, lubricate the bearings with service oil after the thermal washer disinfector stage. Use separate oil canisters for pre-and postdisinfection oiling. Check that the service oil canister has the correct nozzle attachment for the handpiece, and spray service oil once (approximately one second) through the lumen onto a disposable soft paper towel (Figure 7.12). Place the handpiece with the head downwards in a rack to drain off excess oil, ready for the next stage in the decontamination cycle. For thermal washer

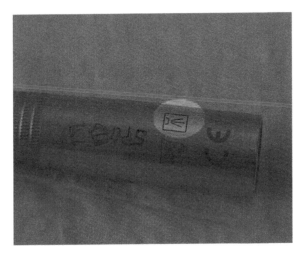

Figure 7.11 Thermal washer disinfector safe symbol on a dental handpiece.

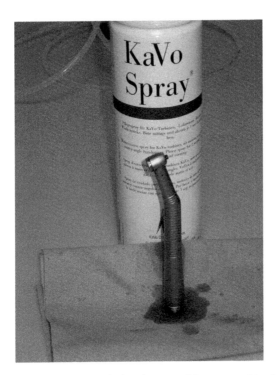

Figure 7.12 Service oil is sprayed into the handpiece and the excess oil is allowed to drain out.

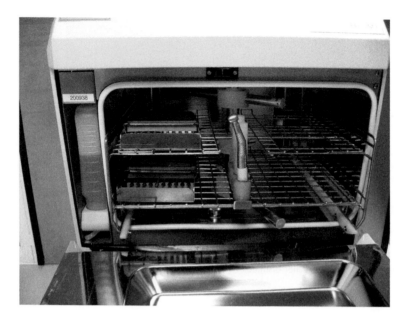

Figure 7.13 Handpiece connectors in a thermal washer disinfector. If the connector is fitted with a filter, these require regular cleaning.

disinfector intolerant handpieces, follow the manufacturer's instruction on disinfection (Figure 7.13).

MECHANICAL CLEANING WITH AN ULTRASONIC BATH

Ultrasonic baths are significantly more effective than manual cleaning.

An ultrasonic cleaner has a variety of functions. An ultrasonic bath can be used as an alternative to manual cleaning when a thermal washer disinfector is unavailable or as a back-up automated cleaning process in the event of thermal washer disinfector failure. They are highly effective at removal of adherent debris such as hardened cements and for cleaning intricate, hinged or jointed and serrated metal, although, ideally, the clinician or nurse should remove cement from dental hand instruments at the chair-side before it sets. Ultrasonic baths are *unsuitable* for cleaning dental handpieces. Plastic instruments are not successfully cleaned in an ultrasonic bath as they absorb the ultrasonic energy.

Ultrasonic cleaning works by cavitation generated by high-frequency sound waves that create regions of alternating high and low pressure in the bath. Bubbles form in the detergent under low-pressure implode when the pressure

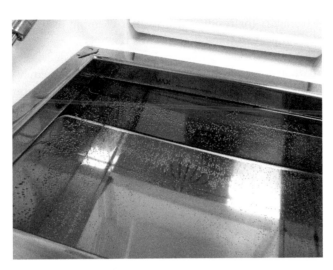

Figure 7.14 The figure shows bubbles of dissolved oxygen in an ultrasonic bath. If not removed, they collect on the surface of the instruments and interfere with the cavitation action of the bath. They are removed by degassing the bath.

changes from low to high, dislodging debris from nooks and crannies and cleaning the surface. Water absorbs oxygen and this is released as bubbles of oxygen gas, which interfere with the cleaning action of the bath (Figure 7.14). To avoid this problem, degas the detergent solution by running the bath empty for a few minutes before immersing the instruments. Removing the oxygen bubbles will improve the efficiency of the cavitation process.

Remember that the ultrasonic baths only clean and remove micro-organisms; they do not disinfect instruments as the running temperature is below the minimum required to kill even vegetative bacteria. Enzymatic cleaners used in ultrasonic baths degrade proteins but may have no disinfection effect on viruses.

Good practice guide: using an ultrasonic bath

- Rinse off blood and gross debris by immersing instruments under warm water. Instruments do not need to be scrubbed before placing in the bath.
- Fill bath with detergent solution. Use the detergent at the concentration recommended by manufacturer. Set bath temperature at below 45 °C or use manufacturer's default temperature setting (this minimizes protein coagulation).
- Place instruments in a basket. Do not place any instruments on the floor of the bath as this can damage the instrument. Open hinged instruments and dismantle multipart instruments.
- At the end of the cycle, rinse instruments thoroughly to remove detergent residues by immersing in clean water (unless machine has an automatic rinse cycle) and dry with a non-linting cloth.

- Inspect instruments for residual debris after cleaning using an illuminated magnifier and repeat cleaning if any debris remains.
- Ultrasonic bath solutions become contaminated with debris, so empty and clean the bath at the end of the clinical session (approximately four hours) or more frequently if the solution becomes visibly heavily contaminated.
- Only operate with the lid closed to avoid aerosol contamination. Some baths have an interlocking device to prevent removal of instruments during the cycle.
- Empty, clean and dry the bath at the end of the day.

Good practice guide: maintenance and validation of ultrasonic bath

- Some baths are fitted with a printer or data-logger to give a retainable record of each cleaning cycle.
- Once weekly, test the cleaning efficiency of the bath using a protein detection test kit (Figure 7.15).
- Undertake a protein residue test once weekly on a random set of instruments to confirm the cleaning *efficiency* of the ultrasonic bath (see Figure 7.10).
- Perform a quarterly *validation test* to confirm the bath is fully functional. Validate with an electronic or commercial test or use the foil ablation test. Use a standard foil manufactured for the test. A series of nine foil strips are suspended in the bath from a grid and the bath is run (Figure 7.16a). Inspect all the foil strips. The edges of each of the foil strips should be serrated with pitting and/or perforation of centre of the strip (Figure 7.16b). Retain the test strips and record the test results as pass or fail in the machine logbook. If the ultrasonic bath fails the test, repeat and if it fails again, stop using the bath and contact the service engineer (Figure 7.16c).
- Get the bath regularly serviced, validated and tested by a suitably qualified engineer (usually annually; see HTM 01-05). All test results and validation should be retained in the ultrasonic bath logbook for a minimum of two years.

THERMAL WASHER DISINFECTORS

> Washer disinfectors provide automated, reproducible and validated cleaning.

Most thermal washer disinfectors have an operating cycle that includes a cool prewash (below 45 °C to prevent protein coagulation and remove debris), main wash, rinse, thermal disinfection and postdisinfection rinse. Thermal disinfection is achieved by the use of hot water (set at 80 °C for 10 minutes or 90 °C for 1 minute; EN ISO Standard 15883) coming into direct contact with the

(a)

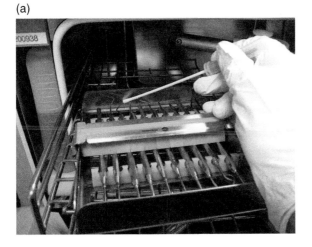

(b)

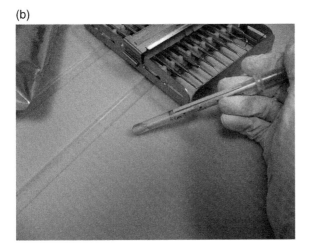

(c)

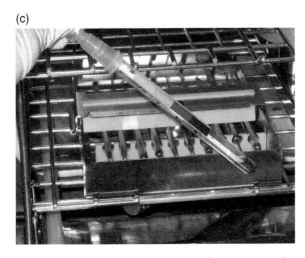

Figure 7.15 Protein detection test. (a) A random set of instruments and tray are swabbed and the swab is inserted into the test solution of ninhydrin. If protein is present the solution will turn blue-purple. (b) A pass test. (c) A fail.

(a)

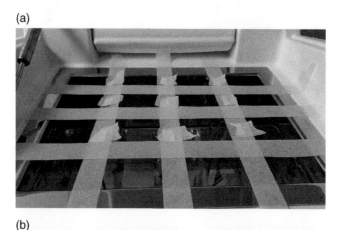

(b)

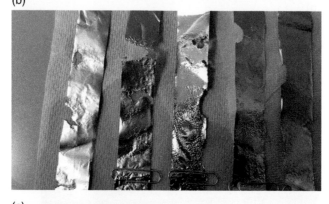

(c)

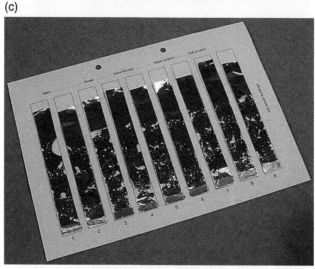

Figure 7.16 Foil ablation test. (a) Nine foil strips suspended from a 3 × 3 grid made from masking tape suspended across the ultrasonic bath. (b) Close-up view demonstrating pitting and perforation of the foil strips indicating that the ultrasonic bath is working satisfactorily. (c) Foil strips mounted on a test sheet, retained as a permanent record in the machine logbook. Source: Courtesy of Paul Jenkins.

instruments and equipment for a specified period of time, followed by a drying cycle. Thermal disinfection reduces the number of viable micro-organisms contaminating the devices, but may not inactivate some viruses and bacterial spores, so instruments are not sterile at the end of the programme. This is followed by a rinse stage which removes residual detergent. Mains water can be used for the rinse water if advised by the manufacturer or a high-quality water such as reverse osmosis (RO) water, which is virtually free of pathogens and endotoxins. In hard-water areas, a water softener is recommended to treat the feed water supply (Figure 7.17). Machines are designed with independent 'watchdog circuits' that monitor the detergent dosing verification, detergent cleaning cycle and thermal disinfection cycle. They are programmed to alert the operator to any failures or malfunctions, and will abort the cycle if errors are detected. An integrated printer or data-logger provides a permanent record of the operation parameters and performance indicators of the disinfection cycle.

Domestic dishwashers are not an acceptable alternative. They do not perform to the same specifications as the washer disinfectors and may not adequately clean the inner surface of hollow or lumened instruments, nor are they capable of validation in accordance with HTM 01-05or BS EN ISO 15883 (Washer Disinfectors).

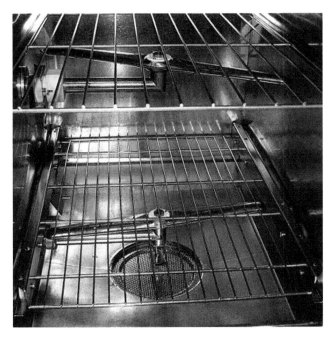

Figure 7.17 Scaling and staining of the interior walls and floor of a thermal washer disinfector which has been connected to an unsuitable water supply; compare the sheen on the horizontal shelf to the staining of the other surfaces. Source: Courtesy of Paul Jenkins.

Multipurpose trays/cassettes are commercially available that are suitable for clinical use in the surgery, the thermal washer disinfector, the sterilizer and for storage, thereby significantly reducing the amount of instrument handling by the nurse, which in turn decreases the incidence of sharps injuries. Trays also aid in instrument stock control.

INSTRUMENT INSPECTION

Instruments should be function tested as part of the decontamination process. Instruments that are damaged should be repaired or taken out of service. Instruments that develop or sustain surface damage due to general wear, pitting or corrosion encourage dirt and bacteria to accumulate and are more difficult to clean effectively. Rusty and corroded instruments cannot be sterilized, as the rust acts as an insulating layer and beneath the rust microbes are afforded protection from the sterilizing temperature. Furthermore, they may be more prone to failing during function and could potentially harm patients or staff.

DENTAL INSTRUMENT STERILIZATION

Sterilization is the stage in the decontamination cycle targeting the killing and removal of microbial contamination, in particular bacterial spores. Invasive instruments that breach the mucosa or intact skin need to be sterile at the point of use in order to prevent wound infection and the transfer of micro-organisms from person to person. Therefore, benchtop steam sterilizers used in the dental practice must be suitable for the intended instrument load, and be validated before use, maintained and operated properly to ensure that the load is sterilized on every occasion.

SUITABILITY OF STERILIZER FOR DIFFERENT LOADS

Never sterilize heat-sensitive items or single-use items in any type of sterilizer.

There are three main types of benchtop sterilizers available for use in dentistry, namely N-type non-vacuum (also known as downward displacement/ gravity displacement) sterilizers and B- and S-type vacuum benchtop sterilizers. The suitability of these three types of sterilizers for different types of equipment is summarized in Table 7.2. Steam sterilization relies on complete air removal in order for the steam to come into intimate contact with the

Table 7.2 Suitability of sterilizers for different types of instruments

Type	Air removal	Suitability for different types of instruments
N	Passive (downward, gravity displacement)	Solid, non-wrapped
B	Active air removal by vacuum pulse	All types of equipment including: hollow (e.g. forceps) lumened (e.g. dental handpieces) wrapped and porous (e.g. swabs)
S	Active air removal by vacuum superatmospheric pulsing; steam injection through lumen	Only suitable for loads specified by manufacturer

entire surface of a device within the chamber. B-type and S-type sterilizers are suitable for hollow and solid instruments as the air is removed actively with the aid of a vacuum phase. A poststerilization drying stage ensures that the load is dry before the door is opened, allowing the instruments to be wrapped or pouched prior to sterilization. However, this prolongs the total cycle time considerably.

A non-vacuum phase sterilizer utilizes gravity and passive displacement of the air by the steam. When used for the sterilization of instruments with lumens, inadequate air removal from the interior of the instrument can occur, which may result in failure to completely sterilize the entire lumen. Unfortunately, cases of serious infection have ensued when such incompletely sterilized instruments were used on vulnerable patients. However, in the UK, national guidelines permit the use of N-type sterilizers to sterilize dental handpieces for routine dentistry even though sterility is not guaranteed, but not for invasive surgical use.

STERILIZER INSTALLATION AND VALIDATION

Before use, a new sterilizer has to be installed, commissioned and validated by an accredited service engineer (also referred to as a 'competent person-decontamination' in the technical literature). The documentation is retained for a minimum of two years in the sterilizer logbook for future reference. All steam sterilizers and associated pipework are subject to the Pressure Systems Safety Regulations 2000 as these can be dangerous items of equipment unless regularly validated and maintained by an accredited engineer (see Chapter 1).

STERILIZATION AND DISINFECTION OF DENTAL INSTRUMENTS

STEAM PURITY AND MAINTENANCE OF WATER RESERVOIR CHAMBER

All sterilizers have a reservoir chamber from which the water is delivered for steam generation. Tap water is not recommended as it contains dissolved minerals, which can cause scaling of the heating element and the chamber, adversely affecting the normal functioning of the sterilizer. The water needs to be of high quality to safeguard both the patient and the sterilizer. As the water cools in the reservoir, the temperatures become suitable for bacterial growth and a bacterial biofilm will form on the walls and floor of the chamber (see Chapter 9 for an explanation of bacterial biofilm formation). In a surveillance study, microbiological sampling of sterilizer reservoirs in dental practices where they were not appropriately maintained revealed a bacterial count of the order of 10^4–10^5 cfu/mL. The bacterial count and associated endotoxin titres in these contaminated sterilizers were virtually eliminated after daily cleaning of the reservoir and refilling with fresh purified water.

Current guidance recommends that sterilizer reservoir water and steam should be 'free of pathogens and endotoxins' (pyrogen), and contain a low specified amount of inorganic minerals. Bacteria in the reservoir water are killed during the steam generation process, but the endotoxins (lipopolysaccharides) released from the bacterial cell walls remain, and as the water in the steam condenses on cooling, it coats the instruments with endotoxins. Bacterial endotoxins are biologically active even when the bacteria from which they are released are dead. Endotoxins cause hypersensitivity reactions, toxic shock, gingivitis and periodontal disease, and can inhibit wound healing.

Types of water and steam purity

Suitable types of water that have the desired properties include sterile water, distilled water and reverse osmosis water. RO water is made by forcing water through a series of semi-permeable membranes under pressure to remove minerals and endotoxins. Bacteria are removed with bacterial filters or ultraviolet light treatment. RO water can be purchased commercially or made on site in the dental surgery. Small on-site RO machines can be plumbed directly into the sterilizer. RO machines need to be maintained and the water periodically sampled and tested for chemical contaminants, mineral content and pH.

Purified waters such as *deionized* or *distilled* waters can also be made in the dental practice. The disadvantage of these types of water is that although they normally have a low mineral content, the actual amount is unknown. They are commonly contaminated with endotoxins and pathogens, but at unspecified levels, so their quality cannot be guaranteed.

Partially used bottles of commercial water or locally produced waters should be discarded at the end of the day as the microbiological quality of all types of water deteriorates rapidly on storage. Bacteria divide approximately every 20 minutes and grow exponentially so, starting with one bacterium in a bottle of water, after a seven-hour working day there will be over 4 million bacteria – a veritable bacterial soup!

Problems associated with recycled water

Depending on the model of sterilizer, water in the reservoir is either recycled or used once and discharged into the drain at the end of the sterilization cycle. Where water is recycled, it will become progressively more contaminated by the end of each cycle with endotoxins and lubricant oil that are then deposited on subsequent instrument loads. Therefore, modern sterilizers were redesigned to employ single-shot water systems to avoid this problem.

Good practice guide: daily maintenance of sterilizer reservoir

- Fill with fresh (commercial or produced on-site) RO water or distilled water. Do not use tap water, which can lead to a build-up of harmful contaminants and limescale.
- Regularly disinfect the RO machine and validate the water quality according to the manufacturer's instructions.
- Allow water to cool and then drain down and replenish water in the reservoir at least daily. Do not top up. Alternatively, use sterilizer with an automated single-use water cycle.
- Dispose of partially used bottles or locally produced water at the end of the day (avoid storage of water for greater than 12 hours).
- At the end of the day, wipe down the reservoir with fresh RO or distilled water, using a disposable non-linting cloth, dried and covered with a lid. Do not use a disinfectant, unless specifically recommended by the manufacturer, as this can damage the pipework.
- Leave reservoir empty until future use.

HOW DO YOU KNOW YOUR STERILIZER IS WORKING?

Periodic testing of the sterilizer

To kill micro-organisms, the instruments need to be exposed to steam at a specified temperature for a specific holding time. Although other options exist, the preferred temperature-pressure-time relationship for all small steam sterilizers is 134–137 °C, 2.1–2.25 bar gauge pressure for at least a three-minute holding time. The automatic controller is the device within the sterilizer that controls the sterilization cycle.

Successful sterilization depends on consistent reproducibility of the sterilizing conditions during every cycle. However, sterilization is a process whose effectiveness cannot be guaranteed by visual inspection or direct, immediate microbiological testing of the sterile product.

In the USA, sterilization is monitored using a combination of biological, mechanical and chemical indicators. Biological indicators, or spore tests, assess the sterilization process's ability to kill highly resistant micro-organisms (e.g. *Geobacillus* or *Bacillus* species). A spore test is recommended to be used at least weekly to monitor sterilizers but because spore tests are only performed periodically and the results are not obtained immediately, mechanical and chemical monitoring is also recommended. Microbiological spore test kits to verify sterilization are not recommended in the UK, as this method cannot provide immediate feedback on sterilizer function and is prone to false-positive results.

In the UK, process monitoring (sometimes referred to as mechanical monitoring) of individual sterilization cycles is the approved method for guaranteeing that instruments and equipment are indeed sterile. This relies on the assumption that if all sterilizing parameters are correct, namely the temperature, pressure and holding time, then the desired outcome, i.e. sterile instruments, will result. Sterilizers fitted with printers or electronic data-loggers will generate this parametric data automatically for each sterilization cycle. At the start of each day, the person responsible for operating the sterilizer checks that the sterilizer is working correctly by running an automatic control test (ACT) and records whether the sterilizer passed or failed the test. This information is recorded in the sterilizer logbook. Each sterilizer in the practice should have its own logbook to record details of the installation, commissioning and validation, and maintenance history, including descriptions of breakdowns and time out of action. All records including the daily ACT should be kept for a minimum of two years according to HTM 01-05.

How to perform the daily automatic control test

The ACT requires the temperature and pressure profiles and the holding time of the cycle to be compared with the values obtained when the sterilizer (vacuum or non-vacuum) was known to be working correctly (i.e. the specific settings for your sterilizer, which were calibrated by the engineer at the most recent validation. These settings will vary slightly for each sterilizer). Perform the ACT using the sterilizing cycle with the highest temperature compatible with the load (usually 134–137 °C) (see Table 7.2). The test is performed either with an empty chamber or with the load composition that is the same each day. If the sterilizer does not have a printer/data-logger fitted, observe the gauges, measure the holding time with a stopwatch and record the following during the sterilizing (holding) stage of the cycle.

- Date and cycle number
- Maximum values of the chamber temperatures and pressures indicated on the gauges
- Holding stage duration in minutes and seconds
- Satisfactory completion of the cycle (absence of failure light)

The most important part of the test is to record in the logbook whether the sterilizer passed or failed the test and this should be signed and dated by the operator. The signature acts as 'a certification of fitness for use'. A lack of operator signature may well be taken by external inspectors to indicate non-compliance.

Test failures

The daily ACT results should be viewed as a medico-legal document; it is the only evidence you have that the sterilizer was working and could protect you from litigation. A failure of the ACT (or steam penetration test described below) indicates that the sterilizer is not working correctly. The practice should have a written procedure for dealing with test failures and the sterilizer should be withdrawn from service until the problem is rectified and a successful test achieved. In addition to the daily ACT, keep the printer readout for every sterilization cycle to provide assurance that sterilized loads are being consistently produced.

Steam penetration test

A vacuum sterilizer, because it has an active vacuum phase, requires additional daily testing in the form of the steam penetration test. This test checks that the vacuum pump is working correctly and the air removal stage is effective and that any residual air and other non-condensable gases (NCGs) will not interfere with the sterilization process. It is essential to perform this test with *only* the steam penetration test device in the chamber. Anything else in the chamber will disrupt the test and produce an erroneous result. Only use the test pack specified by the manufacturer, e.g. Bowie and Dick type (Figure 7.18) or manufacturer's equivalent steam penetration test kit (Helix test; Figure 7.19). Results (pass or fail and the test card) are recorded in the sterilizer logbook and the data kept for a minimum of two years.

(a)

(b)   (c)

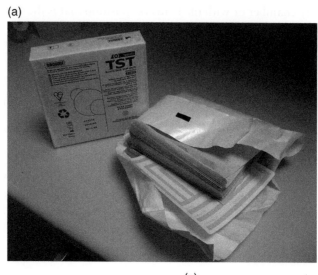
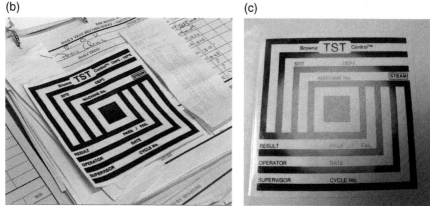

Figure 7.18 (a) A Bowie–Dick test kit showing the yellow test sheet in the centre of the paper pack. (b) A 'pass' Bowie–Dick steam penetration test pasted into the sterilizer logbook. (c) A 'failed' Bowie–Dick test indicating a failure to remove all the air from inside the test pack and replace it with steam, as demonstrated by an incomplete colour change on the indicator sheet.

Chemical process indicators

Chemical process indicators include autoclave tape, test strips, sterilization packaging or pouches printed with a chemical indicator. Typically, chemical monitoring uses sensitive chemicals that change colour when exposed to high temperatures or combinations of time and temperature/steam (multiparameter test strips). These indicators are designed to help you distinguish whether an instrument has been through a sterilizer cycle (Figure 7.20). They offer *no* guarantee that the instrument is sterile. They should not be considered as an alternative to the daily parametric tests, such as the ACT or steam penetration test.

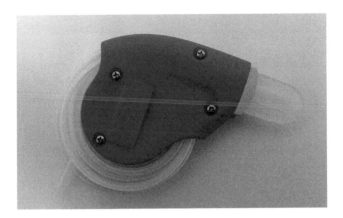

Figure 7.19 Helix test. If the vacuum pump is working correctly, air is withdrawn from the narrow-bore tubing and replaced with steam that penetrates to the indicator test strip, which will change colour.

(a)

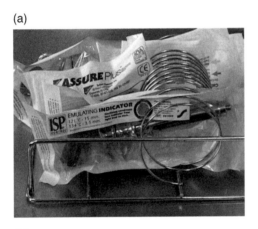

(b)

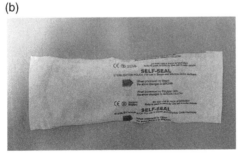

Figure 7.20 (a) Chemical indicator strips inserted within sterilization pouches, which are used to confirm that the pouch has been through a sterilization cycle. They help to differentiate between processed and unprocessed items, eliminating the possibility of using instruments that have not been sterilized. (b) Chemical indicators for steam and ethylene oxide sterilization printed on a self-sealing sterilization pouch.

LOADING THE STERILIZER

The effectiveness of the sterilization process depends upon direct contact between the steam and all surfaces of the load. To sterilize effectively, steam needs to be able to circulate freely. Try to avoid creating trapped air pockets when loading the machine that will prevent the steam making direct contact with the instruments, for example place kidney dishes at an angle so that the air is not trapped inside the bowl. Instruments and equipment are not pouched or wrapped when using non-vacuum sterilizer as this creates an air envelope around the device, which will lower the temperature on the instrument surface and could lead to sterilization failure. Wrapping of instruments or trays is therefore only appropriate for B-type vacuum sterilizers, which can reproducibly remove the trapped air.

Good practice guide: loading the sterilizer

- Instruments should be clean and dry prior to sterilization.
- Sterilizers should never be overloaded; steam should be able to circulate freely. Overloading will also inhibit instrument drying.
- Instruments should be placed across the tray ribs and should not be touching.
- Hinged instruments should be opened.
- Bowls, kidney dishes, etc. should be inverted and placed at an angle to allow draining and the steam to contact all surfaces of the vessel.

STORAGE OF WRAPPED AND UNWRAPPED INSTRUMENTS

Instruments sterilized in a non-vacuum sterilizer for immediate use

After the end of the holding period and sterilizing cycle, the steam condenses in the sterilizer chamber, so the load will be wet unless the sterilizer has a drying cycle. Wet instruments can be used directly from the sterilizer (as the water will be sterile). The sterilized load becomes contaminated with atmospheric bacteria as soon as the chamber door is opened so unwrapped instruments should ideally be used immediately.

It is inadvisable to leave instruments in the sterilizer overnight as condensation can lead to bacterial contamination. Furthermore, confusion can arise as to whether or not instrument sets were processed, especially when several nurses are working together in the decontamination room. If instruments are left inadvertently overnight in the sterilizer before they are used, you should check the printout to see when the sterilization cycle was run and examine the process indicator. If there is any doubt, then resterilize the instruments before use.

Sterile instrument storage

The main purpose of instrument packaging and storage is to prevent microbiological recontamination and packaging degradation and to maintain the sterility of the instruments. Instruments for invasive surgical or dental procedures must be sterile at the point of use, which can only be achieved by prepacking instruments followed by sterilization in a B-type vacuum sterilizer.

Essential practice requirements permit storage of instrument packs in the treatment room in a dedicated drawer or cupboard but this should be as far away as possible from the patient and the dirty zone. Best practice guidelines recommend that sterilized and sterile instrument packs and trays should be stored either in a dedicated clean storage room or a storage area within the clean zone of the decontamination suite. Wherever the sterilized instruments are stored, it must be in a manner that preserves the integrity of the packaging material.

Storage practices can be either date or event related or a combination of the two, as is used in the UK. An event-related approach assumes that a sterilized instrument pack should remain sterile until some event causes the item to become contaminated. A number of studies have shown that sterile packs remain sterile for several years if stored correctly. However, the quality of the packaging material, the conditions under which items are stored and transported, and the amount that they are handled all affect the chances that the package and its contents will remain sterile. All instrument packs should be inspected immediately before use to verify the expiry date, barrier integrity and dryness. Any package that is wet, torn, dropped on the floor or damaged in any way should not be used.

In the UK, the instrument pack is dated with the expiry date. If multiple sterilizers are used in the decontamination suite, then the sterilizer number and the cycle number should be indicated on the outside of the packaging material. This information can facilitate retrieval of processed items in the event of a sterilization failure. Instrument packs can be heat sealed using a device as shown in Figure 7.8, which is fitted with different size rolls of packaging suitable for either instrument trays or single instruments. Self-sealing packs in a variety of sizes are also available commercially.

Always segregate sterile wrapped instruments processed in a B-type vacuum sterilizer from those instruments that are packaged post sterilization, which are sterilized but not sterile. Storage times used in the different countries of the UK are shown in Table 7.3. Unwrapped sterilized items are susceptible to contamination and should be kept in covered trays. Therefore avoid storing items loose in drawers or cabinets; items stored in this manner are subject to contamination from dust, aerosols generated during treatment, and repeated contamination from the hands of personnel who access the drawers to remove instruments.

Storage of unwrapped instruments

Good practice guide: storage of unwrapped instruments

- Sterilized wet instruments should be used immediately.

Table 7.3 Sterilized and sterile instrument storage times*

Non-wrapped instruments sterilized in N-type sterilizer	Wrapped instruments sterilized in vacuum or non-vacuum sterilizer
Store in the surgery: on removal from sterilizer, dry aseptically with non-linting cloth, place in trays or cassettes, cover and use on the same day	**Sterilized in non-vacuum sterilizer**: dry aseptically and wrap in a view pouch* Can be stored for maximum of one year*†
Store in clean zone of the decontamination room: dry aseptically with non-linting cloth, place in trays or cassettes, cover and use within one week*	**Prewrapped in a sterilization pouch and sterilized in a vacuum sterilizer**: can be stored for maximum of one year*

* Storage times recommended by HTM 01-05 – do not apply in Scotland.
† Storage time recommended by the Welsh version WM HTM 01-05; suggests postwrapped instruments can be stored up to one year, but recommends in most cases reprocessing after one month.

- Alternatively, allow instruments to dry in the sterilizer before opening the door. Cover instrument trays or cassettes with a lid or drape and use within the day if kept within the surgery or for one week if stored in a clean storage room. Use stock rotation; when the one-week expiry period is reached, reprocess the instrument through the decontamination cycle
- *Poststerilization wrapping and pouching*: immediately after removal from the sterilizer, dry instruments aseptically using a non-linting disposable cloth; wrap instruments in heat-sealed or self-sealing packs either singly or in trays. Storage for up to one year in a clean dry storage cupboard or drawer is recommended by in HTM 01-05 (see Table 7.3). The instruments will not be sterile but their level of microbial contamination should differ little from those used directly from the sterilizer if kept in a clean and dry condition. Micro-organisms carried in dust particles in the atmosphere are unlikely to proliferate in dry conditions.

Good practice guide: storage of wrapped instruments processed in a vacuum sterilizer

- Wrapped instruments processed in a vacuum autoclave with a drying cycle can be stored for up to 12 months (HTM 01-05) in a clean, dry and dust-free environment. Collection of dust on the packaging may compromise its integrity and reduce the shelf-life.
- If the wrapping or sterilization pouches are wet on removal from the sterilizer or subsequently become wet during storage, the contents will no longer be sterile and will require resterilization.
- Do not attempt to dry damp packages.
- Record the expiry date (date of decontamination, cycle number may also be recorded) on the packaging or pouch.
- Use simple first-in, first-out stock rotation based on the instrument expiry date.
- Keep your standard kits to a minimum. Do not put out instruments you do not need.

Stock control and instrument traceability

Rationalization of the instruments used during routine clinical procedures into standard sets of instruments simplifies and streamlines the decontamination process. In order to aid stock control and for instrument traceability, keep sets of instruments together in the trays or cassettes so that the tray rather than the individual instrument is the unit of tracking. Sophisticated tracking systems that can read barcodes laser printed on individual instruments are in use in sterile service departments, but this type of technology is currently inappropriate in a small dental practice with limited stocks of instruments. An automated label printer linked to the microprocessor in the sterilizer can be programmed to record the cycle number, name of operator, date of decontamination and expiry date and print this information on the label. The peel-off label is then placed in the patient's notes or scanned using a barcode reader into the electronic patient notes (Figure 7.21).

Out-of-hours use of instruments

As described previously, always fully decontaminate instruments as soon as possible after use. However, if a patient is seen late or out of normal working hours, clean and dry instruments at the end of the treatment session. If

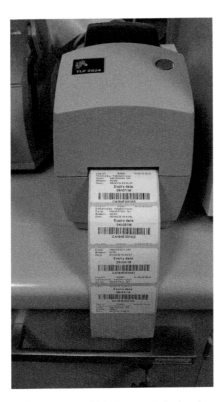

Figure 7.21 An example of an automated label printer linked to the sterilizer microprocessor.

instruments cannot be sterilized, clearly label them as unsafe for handling or use and reprocess them through the full decontamination cycle the next working day.

SINGLE-USE ITEMS

> Never reuse medical devices designated for single use.

A single-use instrument is a medical device that is intended to be used on an individual patient during a single procedure and then discarded. It should not be reused even on the same patient. Instruments and equipment manufactured for single use carry the symbol of a 2 crossed through with a line (Figure 7.22).

The reuse of single-use dental equipment can compromise its safety, performance and effectiveness, exposing patients, clinicians or students to unnecessary risk. By definition, single-use devices have not undergone extensive manufacturer testing and validation to ensure that the device is safe to reuse. Reprocessing a single-use device may alter its characteristics so that plastics become brittle or low-grade metals corrode during sterilization. The device may fail mechanically with reuse due to stress fatigue. Single-use devices are not required to be designed to allow for effective decontamination. Studies have shown that due to the surface defects and pitting of the metal surface of matrix bands, files and reamers, they cannot be successfully decontaminated by

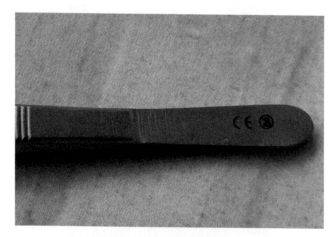

Figure 7.22 International symbol designating 'single-use only' on disposable tweezers. Note the pitting and striations of the metal surface of this single-use item, which would impede any attempts at resterilization.

Box 7.3   Categories of dental equipment best replaced with single-use items

- Hard-to-clean items with narrow lumens: saliva ejectors and suction tips
- Brushes: demonstration toothbrushes, rubber prophy cups and bristle brushes
- Complex intricate devices: stainless steel burs, endodontic files and reamers and plastic impression trays
- Invasive instruments and sharps: matrix bands, scalpels, needles and suture needles

Note: This list is not exhaustive; it contains examples only.

---

cleaning and sterilization. Proteinaceous material which can harbour microbes and prions adheres to the walls of the pits and crevices in the metal surface and is protected from scrubbing brushes and water jets. Other hard-to-clean items include those with narrow lumens and brushes. Hence such items have been replaced with single-use devices (Box 7.3).

If the dentist decides to reuse a single-use item, the product liability for its performance is then transferred from the manufacturer to themselves. This means that the person who reprocesses a single-use device has the same legal obligations and responsibilities under the Medical Devices Regulations as the original manufacturer of the device. If the device after reprocessing is no longer 'fit for the intended purpose' then the dentist may be committing an offence and is at risk of prosecution under both European and UK law.

Quality of single-use instruments

Prompted initially by concerns over the difficulties associated with removing prions from metal instruments but also the problem with effectively cleaning instruments with a narrow lumen in non-vacuum sterilizers, manufacturers have responded by producing a full range of dental instruments in a single-use disposable format. There is a caveat; important lessons were learnt from the wholesale transference to single-use instruments for tonsillectomies, a procedure considered to be high risk for the transmission of vCJD. Unfortunately, the initial design of single-use instruments did not have the same high-performance specification of the standard instruments and tragically a number of deaths occurred because the instruments failed during surgery. Therefore, single-use instruments must be of high quality and demonstrate an equivalent performance standard to their reusable counterparts.

Endodontic files are difficult to clean and should be single use only.

VARIANT CJD AND RATIONALE FOR SINGLE-USE ITEMS

Prions have also been identified in the trigeminal ganglion and tonsils from patients at postmortem and in the dental pulp, gingivae and other oral tissues in animal models. Confirmed reports of CJD transmission occurring iatrogenically due to inadequately decontaminated instruments continue to accumulate and animal model studies have demonstrated vCJD transmission from vCJD-contaminated dental instruments.

Armed with this knowledge, we can make an initial risk assessment of the likelihood of prion transmission occurring during dental treatment. As with all emerging pathogens, our knowledge base continues to evolve as our understanding grows. Abrasion of the lingual tonsil is considered a highly unlikely event during routine dental treatment, but could occur during maxillofacial procedures such as removal of third molars. Dental pulp, which is composed of vascular and peripheral nerve tissue, was shown in animal studies to be infected with vCJD. Similarly, the dental pulp of individuals subclinically infected with vCJD may be infectious, although the level of infectivity is unknown. Appreciable quantities of residual pulp tissue remain adherent to the surface of an endodontic instrument after cleaning and sterilization. A small percentage of endodontic treatments will be carried out on asymptomatic carriers of vCJD. In the UK, over a million endodontic treatments are performed every year. As a result of the large number of treatments, the statistical probability for cross-infection between patients involving contaminated reused endodontic instruments is substantially magnified. As prion-infected carriers move in and out of the dental and medical healthcare systems, every episode of treatment becomes an opportunity for further transmission of vCJD or CJD. Therefore, restricting endodontic files and reamers to single use only at a stroke eliminates this dental route of transmission and with it the potential for ramifications through the rest of the health service.

Furthermore, there are two additional advantages to the designation of endodontic files and reamers as single use. First, the process of sterilization blunts the cutting edge of the file or reamer, hampering its effective use. Second, accidental breakage of an instrument within the root canal is less likely to occur with a single-use instrument. Endodontic files and reamers sold as reusable by the manufacturer can be reused on a single patient following decontamination but only for a multivisit root treatment and then must be disposed of in order to comply with the regulations on single-use instruments.

DISINFECTION OF HEAT-SENSITIVE EQUIPMENT AND HARD SURFACES

In the past, the so-called 'cold sterilization' of routine dental instruments with disinfectants (e.g. glutaraldehyde) was commonly used in dentistry in the UK, but is *no longer* accepted as a mode of instrument sterilization. Nowadays, most dental equipment is manufactured to withstand steam sterilization or, if not, is available as a sterile single-use disposable item. Dental practices should avoid purchasing equipment that cannot be sterilized whenever possible. Therefore, except for *high-level disinfection* of heat-sensitive items of equipment (for example, fibreoptic nasoendoscopes) that cannot be reprocessed by steam sterilization, the use of chemical disinfection is strongly discouraged in dental practice. As a matter of principle, the thermal biocidal action of heat is always preferred to chemicals for disinfection. The reason is that the use of chemicals is more difficult to validate and reproduce and many disinfectants, such as alcohols, are inactivated by the presence of organic matter. In sterile service departments in the acute sector, such heat-sensitive items may be treated with ethylene oxide or hydrogen peroxide gas plasma to achieve sterility.

Glutaraldehyde went out of favour in the UK as a disinfectant because it is a potent irritant and sensitizes the skin, eyes and respiratory tract. Alternative, non-gluteraldehyde containing products are sold for high-level disinfection and are composed of chemicals such as ortho-phthalaldehydes, peracetic acid and hydrogen peroxide. In the USA, the FDA permits the use of glutaraldehyde and distinguishes between high-level disinfection and cold sterilization, depending on the duration of the immersion time. Products sold as sterilants may require immersion for up to 10 hours whereas high-level disinfection takes between 10–45 minutes, depending on the product.

Box 7.4 shows the ideal properties for chemical disinfectants for disinfection of dental impressions or hard surfaces (e.g. bracket tables and worktops). Always select a disinfectant that is compatible with the item and will not damage the surface or have a deleterious effect on its function and follow the manufacturer's instructions for its use. Health and safety legislation requires that a COSHH risk assessment is prepared for all disinfectants used in dental practice; this is normally derived from data supplied in the manufacturer's safety

---

Box 7.4   Ideal properties for a general-purpose hard surface dental disinfectant

- Non-toxic
- Non-allergenic
- Non-irritant
- Non-corrosive
- Does not leave a residue
- Wide range of antimicrobial activity (including killing or destruction of bacterial spores, *Mycobacterium tuberculosis* and viruses including HIV, HCV and HBV)
- Short contact time
- Not inactivated by organic material
- Has a long shelf-life
- Carries a CE mark and is supplied with a manufacturer's safety data sheet

HBV, hepatitis B virus; HCV, hepatitis C virus; HIV, human immunodeficiency virus.

data sheet. See Tables A.2 and A.3 in the Appendix for a description of the types of disinfectants suitable for use in the dental surgery and methods for disinfecting specific items of equipment.

DISINFECTION OF DENTAL IMPRESSIONS

When taking an impression of the teeth or an edentulous ridge, the impression material will become contaminated with saliva, blood, oral micro-organisms and coughed-up respiratory pathogens. Impressions taken on patients with active tuberculosis were found to harbour *Mycobacterium tuberculosis*.

Method for disinfection of dental impressions

- Clean and disinfect all impressions before they are sent to the laboratory.
- Wear gloves, mask, goggles/face shield.
- Thoroughly rinse all impressions in running water to remove all visible signs of contamination.
- Choose a disinfectant that is compatible with impression material. Make up a fresh solution or check that the existing solution is within its use-by date. Pour the solution into a clean container with a secure lid.
- Immerse the impression in the disinfectant for the specified time. Avoid spray disinfectants, which are less effective at penetrating the complex surface of the impression and may create an inhalation risk.
- Rinse off the disinfectant with water.

Commercially manufactured plastic impression trays are destined for single patient use only and should be disposed of as hazardous clinical waste by the practice or the dental laboratory. Metal impression trays are reusable and should be thoroughly cleaned, preferably in a thermal washer disinfector or alternatively in an ultrasonic bath, and then steam sterilized.

REFERENCES AND WEBSITES

Centers for Disease Control and Prevention. Summary of Infection Prevention Practices in Dental Settings: Basic Expectations for Safe Care. Available at: www.cdc.gov/oralhealth/infectioncontrol/pdf/safe-care.pdf (accessed 1 November 2016).

Department of Health. Decontamination in Primary Care Dental Practices (HTM 01-05). Available at: www.gov.uk/government/publications/decontamination-in-primary-care-dental-practices (accessed 1 November 2016).

Medicines and Healthcare products Regulatory Agency. Single-Use Medical Devices: Implications and Consequences of Reuse. Available at: www.gov.uk/government/

publications/single-use-medical-devices-implications-and-consequences-of-re-use (accessed 1 November 2016).

Scottish Dental Clinical Effectiveness Programme. Decontamination into Practice. Available at: www.sdcep.org.uk/published-guidance/decontamination/(accessed 1 November 2016).

Walker JT, Dickinson J, Sutton J.M, Raven NDH, Marsh PD. (2007) Cleanability of dental instruments: implications of residual protein and risks from Creutzfeldt–Jakob disease. *British Dental Journal*, 203, 395–401.

Chapter 8

Dental surgery design, surface decontamination and managing aerosols

DENTAL SURGERY DESIGN

Design and layout of a dental surgery/office should be suitable for carrying out dental services and should promote infection control and prevention. A successful design can make the built environment look stylish and attractive and if appropriate, can facilitate cleanliness and ease of cleaning. People's behaviour can be both positively and negatively influenced by the design of the surgery. Appropriate design features can encourage hand hygiene, help avoid contamination of surfaces and promote tidiness. Therefore, the dental surgery/office should be laid out so that it has sufficient space for the dental team to work, with adequate storage space, lighting, ventilation and temperature control. Overall, the practice environment should look and be uncluttered, clean, dry, well lit and well ventilated.

All fittings and finishes in dentistry should be chosen with cleaning and disinfection in mind (i.e. be smooth, non-porous and water resistant), especially those where contamination with blood or body fluids is a possibility. Maintenance is critically important in the prevention and control of infection, avoiding cracks and tears in finishes where dirt and biofilms can build up. High-quality finishes, fixtures and fittings often require less maintenance over their lifespan and are better able to withstand heavy usage and repeated cleaning with disinfectants.

A well-designed practice provides not only a pleasant working environment for the team but also one that is welcoming and increases patient confidence that the practice is a safe and professional place to visit. First impressions are all-important. In the following section, we have explained in brief the design features and layout in the dental surgery/office, that incorporate a risk-based

Basic Guide to Infection Prevention and Control in Dentistry, Second Edition.
Caroline L. Pankhurst.
© 2017 John Wiley & Sons Ltd. Published 2017 by John Wiley & Sons Ltd.
Companion website: www.wiley.com/go/pankhurst/infection-prevention

approach to counteract the routes of transmission of infection discussed in Chapter 2. For those readers who require detailed planning guidance, this can be found in the Health Building Notes cited in the further reading list on the companion website www.wiley.com/go/pankhurst/infection-prevention.

Room size

The dental surgery/office should be of sufficient size to allow ready access to the dental chair and to perform procedures unhindered (typical size: 17m^2). The surgery design should facilitate environmental cleaning and reduce the risk of cross-contamination (see Zoning of work areas, below). Spacing should take into account the amount of and easy access to dental equipment and movement around the dental chair and access for staff to clinical hand basins, storage cupboards, keyboards and screens. When planning the surgery, incorporate into the design ready access for disabled people and wheelchairs that maintain their dignity, not forgetting additional access space around the dental chair needed in case of a medical emergency.

Work surfaces and zoning

- Areas within clean and dirty 'zones' for practice should be clearly identified to reduce the risk of cross-contamination (Figure 8.1).
- The room should be uncluttered to allow easy access for cleaning.
- Work surfaces should be easy to clean, which can be achieved by using finishes that are impervious, smooth and seamless, as far as practicable. and, wherever possible, curve up at the wall to avoid sharp, difficult-to-clean corners.

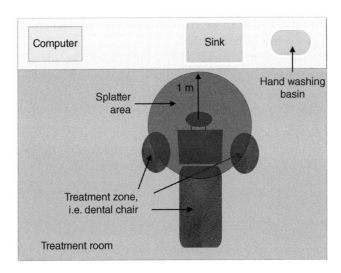

Figure 8.1 Zones within the dental surgery where contamination is likely to occur.

Flooring

- In clinical areas, flooring should be seamless and smooth, slip-resistant, easily cleaned and appropriately wear-resistant.
- Run hard flooring up the walls for a short distance to provide an easy-to-clean coving.
- Any joints should be welded or sealed to prevent accumulation of dirt and damage due to water ingress, blood/body fluid spillages or amalgam/mercury spillages.
- Carpets are *not* permitted in clinical areas. They are hard to keep clean and fragrant in high traffic areas, especially where there is the additional risk of spillages. Carpets cannot be reliably disinfected if contaminated with blood or vomit. Bacteria and fungi have been found growing in carpets in surgeries.

Walls

- Surgery walls should be smooth, cleansable and impervious.
- The finish should be able to withstand the use of detergents and disinfectants and dry quickly when cleaned.
- Additional protection to the walls should be considered to guard against gouging/impacts during daily use. Wall surfaces should be maintained so that they are free from fissures and crevices, which can harbour microbes and are difficult to clean.

Soft furnishings

- Seating used within the surgery and waiting area should be chosen for ease of cleaning and compatibility with detergents and disinfectants.
- Seats are recommended to be covered in a material that is impermeable, preferably seam-free or heat-sealed.
- Soft fabric that becomes soiled and stained cannot be adequately cleaned and will require replacement.

Dental chair

- Dental chairs should be impermeable, intact and easy to wipe down. Chairs should have smooth seamless joins in the covering and on the control panels, which facilitates rapid cleaning and avoids build-up of microbial contamination.

Lighting

- Lighting should be of a suitable construction that allows easy cleaning and does not allow a build-up of dust.
- Lighting used for patient examination must be fitted with a heat filter.

- Handles should be covered with disposable plastic covers, which are replaced between patients.
- Consider hands-free operation of room lighting, e.g. movement sensor automated lights.

Hand basins and hand hygiene

- An easily accessible hand basin should be available in the room, with sensor or lever elbow-operated thermal mixer taps to prevent contamination of the tap. The taps should supply both hot and cold water. Hands should always be washed under running water; the fitting of thermal mixer taps allows this to be carried out safely in dentistry where water temperatures are set at a high level to prevent Legionellae contamination. Aerators and flow restrictors should not be used as they become colonized with bacteria.
- The basin should be specifically dedicated for hand washing and not used for cleaning or storing instruments or disposal of body fluids or chemicals. The hand basin should be large enough to contain most splashes and therefore encourage the correct hand-washing technique as described in Chapter 5 to be performed without splashing the user or their clothing. Wall-mounted taps, if they are placed too high above the sink, will also cause splashing and thereby discourage use and hand hygiene.
- Wash-hand basins should be wall mounted using concealed brackets and fixings. They should also be sealed to a waterproof splash-back to allow effective cleaning of all surfaces.
- Hand-washing sinks should not be fitted with plugs or overflows which are difficult to clean and become contaminated (Figure 8.2).

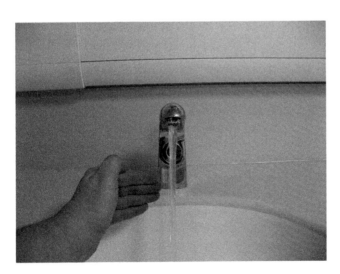

Figure 8.2 Sensor-operated tap fitted on a handwash basin; note there is no overflow.

- The water jet from the tap must not flow directly into the plughole, in order to avoid contamination of the tap with pathogens found in the biofilm that forms in the drain.
- Fit wall-mounted dispensers of rubs or soap solutions that are designed to be operated without contamination from the user's hands coming into direct contact with the dispensing mechanism, i.e. sensor or elbow operated.
- Wall-mounted dispensers of absorbent disposable paper towels should be provided. Paper towels in rolls should be discouraged; they are difficult to tear off without contaminating the remaining roll.
- Under-usage of basins encourages colonization with Legionellae and other micro-organisms due to stagnation. So a balance needs to be struck between ease of access and underuse when designing a dental surgery. Taps on sinks that are infrequently used should be flushed regularly.
- Eliminate or minimize dead-legs and blind ends in water systems, both in the original design and as the plumbing systems are modified over time.
- Supply pipework should be concealed.

Clinical waste sacks and sharps containers

- A foot- or sensor-operated clinical waste sack holder should be conveniently located in the room (see Chapter 10).
- An approved sharps container correctly assembled should be located within easy reach of the clinician, but out of the reach of unauthorized persons and children. It is recommended to wall mount the container or place it in a sturdy base to prevent spillages.

Sharps containers should never be placed on the floor.

Storage of equipment and chemicals

- There should be adequate storage facilities to enable the treatment room and decontamination room(s) to remain uncluttered and ensure that work surfaces are readily accessible and easy to clean.
- Lockable cupboard(s) should be available to store medicines/disinfectants/ chemicals in accordance with Control of Substances Hazardous to Health (COSHH) 2002 Regulations.
- Sterile stock should be stored on covered shelving in a secure, cool, dry and clean environment in order to maintain the integrity of the sterile product and its packaging. (See Chapter 7 for detailed instruction on storage of reusable dental instruments.) Shelving should be readily cleanable and allow for free movement of air around the stored product. Stock should not be stored on the floor.

- Personal belongings should be kept in a separate room.
- Food and drinks should not be consumed in the clinical area.

Ventilation

- Rooms should be well ventilated (open window) or air conditioned. Natural ventilation should not be considered where air circulation could jeopardize cross-infection controls, for example in the decontamination room.
- The recommended fresh air supply rate should not be <5–8 L/second per occupant (approximately 12–15 air changes per hour). However, the means of ventilation should not create uncomfortable draughts.
- Air-cooled air conditioning is preferred to water cooled; any filters should be replaced regularly.
- Ventilation systems should exhaust to the outside of the building but away from places where people congregate, such as bus stops outside high street dental practices.
- Avoid using free-standing or desktop mechanical fans if possible as they circulate dust, splatter and aerosols around the surgery.

Protective clothing

- Provision of storage cupboards and ready access to clean PPE (disposable gloves, plastic aprons, masks and protective eyewear). Personal belongings should be kept in a separate room.

> Do not eat or drink in the patient treatment area. Store food and drinks in a separate fridge from medicines and dental materials.

SURVIVAL OF MICROBES ON SURGERY SURFACES

Surface decontamination of the dental practice (environmental hygiene), like hand hygiene, is an essential tool in breaking the chain of infection. Surface decontamination in the healthcare environment was demonstrated to be key in controlling healthcare-acquired infections (HCAI) caused by Gram-positive pathogens such as methicillin-resistant *Staphylococcus aureus* (MRSA), vancomycin-resistant enterococci and *Clostridium difficile*. If not removed and destroyed by surface decontamination, MRSA will survive for a year in dust, the spores of *C. difficile* for five months and vancomycin-resistant enterococci for four months. Different species of bacteria have adapted to specific niches. Dust-loving *A. baumannii* settles on rarely cleaned and/or inaccessible surfaces such as shelves, highly placed equipment and computer keyboards whereas coliforms such as *Klebsiella* and *Serratia* favour buckets, bowls, mops and liquids over dry surfaces. Some Gram-negative pathogens, notably *Pseudomonas* spp., can survive well in a variety of habitats, normally showing a predilection for damp places such as taps, showers and sinks. Yet they can survive on dry floors for five weeks (see Chapter 9 for the management of *Pseudomonas* spp. in dental plumbing).

Patients and staff become colonized by the microbes in their immediate environment. In hospitals, it has been demonstrated that if the patient who had the room previously was colonized or infected with a Gram-negative pathogen, then there is a high risk that the next patient to stay in the room will also become colonized or infected with the same bacteria. In dentistry, the noses of dental staff become colonized by Gram-negative bacteria found growing in the dental unit waterlines. So we can see that maintaining a clean environment in the dental practice is not just about aesthetics and social norms but is an essential component of infection prevention and control. In England, dental practice cleanliness is a CQC registration requirement (see Chapter 1).

GENERAL CLEANING

Cleaning plan

National cleaning guidelines state that a dental practice must appoint a nominated person to oversee that cleaning requirements are identified, risks are assessed, and cleaning is allocated to the appropriate person and meets the required standard. To ensure the quality of the cleaning services and identify any shortcomings, the nominated person should inspect and audit the cleaning undertaken in the dental premises. As part of the practice's suite of infection control policies, there should be a written protocol (cleaning plan) outlining the cleaning schedule and responsibilities for cleaning the clinical and non-clinical areas (domestic cleaning). Domestic cleaning staff are trained according to the schedule in the cleaning plan (Table 8.1). Logically, high-risk areas are cleaned more frequently within the surgery and decontamination room and this should be undertaken by dental nurses who understand the risks. Any domestic cleaner who has contact with body fluids or hazardous clinical waste should be vaccinated against hepatitis B. As a general principle, all floors, rooms and corridors within the practice should be cleaned and damp-dusted daily.

Detergents (preferably CE marked for clinical use) and warm water are adequate for most domestic cleaning requirements, as cleaning, unlike disinfection, is the physical removal of soil, dirt or dust from surfaces. Use of disinfectants should be restricted to cleaning in the dirty zone where bactericidal activity is required. Overuse of disinfectant is to be avoided, as bacterial resistance mechanisms to disinfectants are often present on the same genetic elements as those conferring resistance to antibiotics, resulting in inadvertent

Table 8.1 An example of a cleaning schedule for a dental practice

Site	Cleaning schedule
Clinical and high-risk areas Carried out by trained members of the clinical team	**Between patients:** clean and disinfect surfaces and equipment used in the 'dirty zone' using single-use disposable disinfectant wipes
	At the end of each clinical session: clean and disinfect all equipment, surfaces within clean and dirty zones used during the treatment of patients using single-use disposable disinfectant wipes
	Instrument decontamination area/room: surfaces and equipment should be cleaned thoroughly before and after each decontamination cycle
Domestic cleaning Carried out by trained domestic cleaning staff	**Daily:** all rooms and corridors within the practice should be cleaned and damp-dusted, including floors, cupboard doors and other exposed surfaces
	Weekly: clean window blinds, accessible ventilation fittings, shelving, radiators and shelves in cupboards

selection of antibiotic resistance in environmental bacteria and human pathogens. A clean microfibre cloth and water is an alternative cleaning method to cleaning with a cloth and detergent.

Microfibre cloths

Microfibre cloths consist of a vast number of very fine fibres providing an enormous surface area that removes and traps dirt and microbes. The cloth performs either wet or dry without detergents and disinfectants. They are widely employed in hospitals for environmental cleaning. The used cloth is potentially infectious as it is covered in microbes; cloths are laundered in a washing machine at 60–90 °C to remove and destroy the pathogens. Although in studies microfibre cloths have been shown to be highly effective, few dental practices have an on-site washing machine available to launder the cloths, thereby limiting their use in dentistry.

Colour coding of cleaning materials

Cleaning cloths and mops should be used and stored in such a way that they do not recontaminate cleaned surfaces. Cleaning cloths and contaminated cleaning equipment can become a source for spreading pathogens. Bacteria adhere more strongly to damp cloths and mops, and trapped organic material (dirt) on cloths and mops both protects and encourages bacterial growth. Contaminated cleaning equipment has been implicated in hospital outbreaks of infection. Therefore, cloths and mops used to clean higher risk, more heavily contaminated patient treatment areas should be separated from those used to clean lower risk, non-clinical sites such as the reception area. In order to

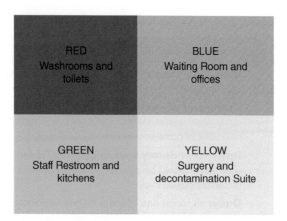

Figure 8.3 National cleaning colour code designations by room.

prevent cross-contamination and simplify the training of domestic cleaning staff, colour coding of cleaning materials, e.g. mops, cloths and buckets, according to the room where they are to be used is recommended (Figure 8.3).

Storage of cleaning materials

The practice should store all cleaning equipment in a clean and dry state. Mop heads should be washed and dried before reuse. Stored buckets, mops and cloths are separated according to their colour code and room designation. It is recommended that they are replaced regularly. An audit trail in the form of simple records to confirm that cleaning has been carried out by the cleaning staff in accordance with the written schedule should be kept as evidence that the dental practice is complying with national cleanliness standards (see Chapter 1). Visual inspection is all that is required in dentistry. In acute healthcare settings, more sensitive indicators of cleanliness are recommended, based on direct sampling to measure the microbial burden on cleaned surfaces or indirect methods such as adenosine triphosphate (ATP) contamination, a surrogate measure of the surface colony count. Interpretation of ATP test results can be problematic, as the relationships between ATP and aerobic colony counts are not necessarily consistent, nor can the test distinguish between harmless environmental species and pathogens.

SURFACE DECONTAMINATION IN THE DENTAL SURGERY

The area around the dental unit becomes contaminated by direct splatter, by droplet nuclei and by touching surfaces with gloved hands. Surface decontamination which embraces both cleaning and disinfection prevents transmission of infection by direct contact with hands and equipment. The reverse is also true, that hand hygiene prevents transmission of surface contaminants. Dental chair, dental handpiece unit, 3-in-1 syringe handle and hoses, lights, bracket table and cabinets, all will require surface decontamination. It is important to train yourself to avoid touching and thereby contaminating drawer handles, pens, computer keyboards and door handles with your gloved hands; it is best to think of these as 'no-touch' surfaces.

Zoning of work areas

Zoning simplifies and streamlines the decontamination process. Its purpose is to distinguish highly contaminated surfaces and work areas, so-called 'dirty zones' (i.e. contaminated by direct contact or splatter during treatment procedures), that require cleaning and disinfection between every patient.

The remaining surgery surfaces are considered to be less likely to be directly contaminated with splatter or by direct contact, but will still have some degree of contamination and therefore must be cleaned at the end of the session and are referred to as the 'clean zone'. Surfaces should be cleaned and disinfected as soon as possible after contamination, as viruses and microbes in surface-dried smears are more resistant to disinfectants. Figure 8.4 shows the areas within the 'dirty zone', which require disinfection between patients. Cleaning is more

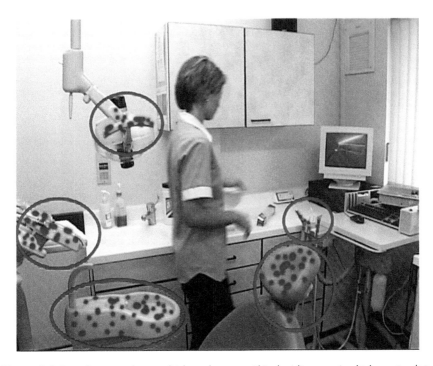

Figure 8.4 Dental surgery showing high-touch areas within the 'dirty zone', which require disinfection between every patient.

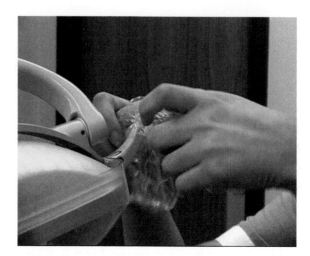

Figure 8.5 Covering a light handle with plastic wrapping.

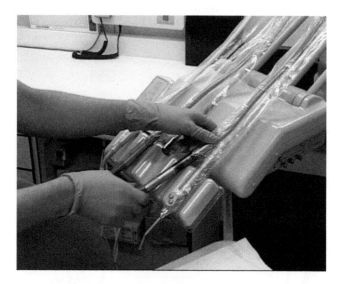

Figure 8.6 Covering areas that are difficult to disinfect with plastic sleeves.

effective in preventing cross-contamination if the most heavily contaminated areas are cleaned first, so begin with cleaning the dirty zone.

Spray disinfectants are discouraged as they can lead to asthma and hypersensitivity reactions and have been replaced with wipes. For surface cleaning, choose a wipe that has dual detergent and disinfectant activity, that has a short contact time and is cidal against oral, skin, pulmonary and environmental bacterial and viruses, and dries to leave no or a minimal surface residue.

The disinfectant wipe should be used in a single direction – a circular wiping motion is not recommended as this will reinfect the area that has just been cleaned.

Single-use disposable plastic sleeves and sheets are used to aid cleaning of high-touch (Figures 8.5 and 8.6) or difficult-to-clean components such as switches, light handles, buttons on 3-in-1, ultrasonic handle, control buttons on the dental chair and headrests. Covers should be removed and the underlying surfaces cleaned between each patient.

> The 'dirty zones' or visibly soiled areas must be cleaned and disinfected between each patient.

At the end of each clinical session, all work surfaces, whether within the clean or dirty zones, including taps, drainage points, splash-backs and sinks, need to be thoroughly cleaned and disinfected using a disposable disinfectant wipe. Key points for zoning and surface cleaning are summarized in Box 8.1.

The reduction in micro-organisms achieved by disinfection is only transient, which is why it has to be repeated throughout the working day. A number of innovations in surface decontamination in healthcare settings have tried to

---

Box 8.1   Key points for zoning and surface cleaning

- Dirty zones (likely to be contaminated during dental treatment) should be separated from clean zones.
- Clean zones: cabinets, surgery drawers, radiographs and patients' notes, computer keyboards are clean zones and should *not be touched* with contaminated gloved hands or instruments.
- During patient treatment, impervious clinical sheets or plastic sheaves simplify the cleaning of switches, dials and high-touch contaminated items between patients.
- Items can be passed into 'dirty zones' but contaminated items should not be passed out into 'clean zones'.
- Storage containers of dental materials should not be placed in the 'dirty zone'.
- Impervious clinical sheets or plastic sheaves should be removed and 'dirty zones' disinfected between patients.
- At the end of a working session, all surfaces in dirty and clean zones should be thoroughly cleaned and disinfected with a disinfectant wipe.
- Work surfaces should be kept uncluttered during the day and clear overnight.
- Trap filters must be removed and cleaned on a regular basis (preferably every night), and rinsed thoroughly before being replaced. Bleach or hypochlorite should not be used as they rust metal. Replace according to manufacturer's instructions.

address this issue and improve the efficacy of decontamination. Experimental studies conducted in clinical environments demonstrated significant reductions in microbial burden of between 80% and 90% on high-touch surfaces coated with metallic copper and/or its alloys compared with similar non-copper surfaces. Finishes and fabrics containing copper are commercially available.

Computer equipment

Computer keyboards are best placed whenever possible in the clean zone. Studies have shown that microbes are recovered from 33–95% of keyboards at concentrations high enough to act as vectors for cross-transmission of infection by hands. Guidelines recommend that surgeries should have washable keyboards or use keyboard covers that facilitate daily disinfection or more often if the keyboard is visibly soiled (Figure 8.7). Conventional keyboards can be replaced with easy-to-clean, fully submergible washable versions that can withstand disinfection even with chlorine (Figure 8.8). Pens are readily contaminated in the clinical environment and have long been recognized as a vehicle for transmission of MRSA.

> Disinfectant wipes are preferred to spray-on products because of the generation of unnecessary aerosols, which may cause sensitization of staff and patients.

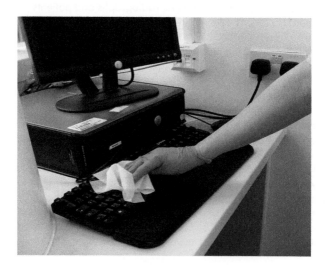

Figure 8.7 Cleaning the keyboard with a disinfectant wipe.

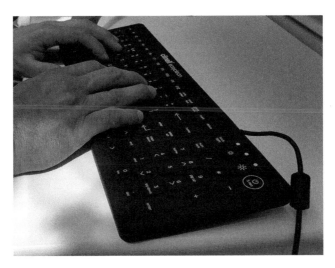

Figure 8.8 An example of a fully submersible washable keyboard.

Managing aspirators, suction apparatus and spittoons

These require special attention as they become grossly contaminated and may be difficult to decontaminate.

- *Spittoons* – clean the outer surface first with a disinfectant wipe and then the inner surface of the bowl, add a (metered) dose of non-foaming disinfectant and then wipe evenly around the inside of the bowl. Leave the disinfectant solution for the contact time required for it to destroy micro-organisms. The time interval is specified by the manufacturer for their product. Then rinse, using the bowl flush, and discard the used disinfection wipe.
- *Aspirators* – flush suction apparatus, drains and spittoons with a non-foaming disinfectant/detergent and leave overnight or according to the manufacturer's instructions (Figure 8.9).

Saliva ejectors

Saliva ejectors are prone to backflow during use and the contents could potentially be expelled into the patient's mouth. Backflow can happen under the following circumstances.

- If the patient sucks or closes his or her lips around the saliva ejector, pressure in the patient's mouth is less than that in the saliva ejector and a partial vacuum is formed, resulting in the backflow of previously aspirated fluids.
- When a reversal of pressure is created as the suction tubing is elevated above the patient's mouth. Care should be taken to ensure that the suction tip and

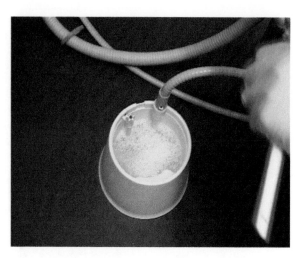

Figure 8.9 Flushing of aspirator suction apparatus with detergent/disinfectant.

line are held below the patient's mouth at all times so that gravity enhances the removal of oral fluids.
- When the high-volume suction is switched on in other parts of the suction system in either the same or adjacent surgeries.

Fortunately, to date there are no documented cases of infection that have been directly linked to backflow from saliva ejectors. However, members of the dental team should be made aware of the small but potential risk of cross-infection associated with saliva ejectors if they are not handled correctly.

MANAGEMENT OF AEROSOLS AND SPLATTER

Splatter, sneezing, coughing and aerosols generated by rotary instruments produce air-borne particles, which vary greatly in size from 0.001 to 10 000 μm. Larger particles or water droplets with a diameter greater than 100 μm are referred to as splatter. Splatter particles travel through the air for a few seconds and then settle within a radius of 1–2 m from the source. Particles in this size bracket are generated by the conventional speed handpiece, air and water syringe and hand basin tap. Surface cleaning and disinfection remove particulates that have settled out and deposited on equipment and work surfaces. Droplets generated during coughing and sneezing consist of air-borne particles between 20 and 100 μm. These can contain large numbers of microbes. Droplets with a particle size less than 20 μm will remain air borne for many minutes, whereas particles greater than 20 μm fall from air-borne suspension within seconds. True aerosols comprise very small particles less than 5 μm or droplet nuclei (fluid droplets that evaporate and shrink to less than $5\,\mu m$) that are capable of remaining in the air for several hours and of travelling long distances on air currents such as out into the waiting room.

Aerosols are generated by a wide variety of dental procedures including, amongst others, the use of high-speed dental handpieces and ultrasonic instrumentation. Coolant dental unit water mixes with blood, saliva, tooth tissue and oral bacteria to produce a contaminated aerosol that can be inhaled into the respiratory passages or deposited on the skin and mucous membranes of the eyes and mouth. Using air sampling techniques, bacterial counts of $>1000\,cfu/m^2/hour$ at $1.5\,m$ distance from the patient have been recorded (Bennett *et al.*, 2000). Ultrasonic scaling produces the highest concentrations of microbes in the aerosol, with peak concentrations recovered approximately 6–12 inches from the operator.

Control of aerosols and splatter

Aspirators remove approximately 90% of the coolant spray (Figure 8.10). Airborne particulates generated during dental treatment have been shown (Rautemaa *et al.*, 2006) to decrease to background levels within 10–30 minutes, due to the rapid deposition of particles at approximately $1\,m$ from the ground or height of the patient's head (see Figure 8.1). The rate of clearance of aerosols in an enclosed space such as a dental surgery is dependent on the ventilation; the greater the number of air changes per hour (ventilation rate), the faster any aerosols will be diluted. Assuming perfect mixing, a single air change removes approximately 63% of air-borne contamination and each subsequent air change removes 63% of what remains; therefore five air changes reduce

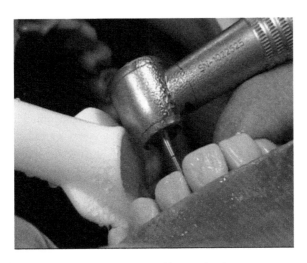

Figure 8.10 Aspirator removing spray generated by an air rotor.

contamination to <1% of its former level. This calculation assumes that further dispersal has ceased. There is no specific number of air changes per hour recommended for dentistry but a minimum figure of 12–15 air changes per hour would be reasonable.

Containment of aerosols is important, as respiratory infections are spread by aerosols and droplets (as discussed in Chapter 2). Methods to reduce the risk of occupational infection involve a combination of aerosol control, ventilation of the surgery, use of PPE and immunization. Aerosol contamination of the surgery can be minimized by the use of:

- high-volume suction (Figure 8.10)
- rubber dam
- proper patient positioning
- rinsing with chlorhexidine mouthwash before scaling (reduces aerosol contamination for approximately 40 minutes after rinsing).

Blood can be recovered from saliva samples after many routine dental procedures (e.g. ultrasonic scaling, orthodontic debonding) even if it is not visible to the naked eye. HIV can be transmitted following splatter exposure of mucous membranes, although the risk of seroconversion is very much lower than that after a needlestick injury. However, there is no published evidence of a blood-borne pathogen being transmitted by aerosol-generating dental procedures.

> Routine use of masks, goggles and visors by dentists, hygienists/therapists and dental nurses will reduce the risks of infection associated with splatter and aerosol.

MANAGING LARGE BLOOD OR BODY FLUID SPILLAGES

Blood and body fluid spillages must be dealt with immediately by trained clinical staff. The size of the spill (spot, small (<30 mL) or large spill) will determine the management. The majority of blood and body fluid spills in the dental surgery are likely to be spots and splashes. Chlorine-releasing granules (e.g. sodium hypochlorite/sodium dichloroisocyanurate) or a liquid solution of hypochlorite at a concentration of 10 000 ppm (1%) should be used for small and large spills, respectively. These should not be added to hot water or mixed with anionic detergents, as this can result in the release of chlorine gas. Disposable gloves, masks and plastic aprons should be worn. (Use eye protection visor/goggles if splashing is likely.) Vomiting may be due to a viral infection, so vomit should be covered immediately with paper towel to prevent aerosolization and spread of virus particles. Body fluid-splattered soft furnishings which cannot withstand chlorine-releasing agents should be subject to a blood-borne virus risk assessment prior to decontamination, and cleaned with a solution of detergent and tepid water. If blood soiling has occurred and soft furnishings cannot be adequately decontaminated then they should be disposed of.

Splashes and spots

- Wear disposable gloves (use masks and plastic aprons if using hypochlorite, and use eye protection visor/goggles if splashing is likely).
- If the surface is non-porous and compatible with hypochlorite, wipe the area with a disposable chlorine wipe (equivalent to 1000 ppm or 0.1% free chlorine).
- Rinse off with clean water and detergent to avoid corrosion or bleaching of the surface.
- Clean area with water and detergent.
- Dry the surface with disposable paper towels.
- Discard gloves, wipe, paper towels as hazardous infectious clinical waste.
- Wash and dry hands.

Small spills (<30 mL)

- Wear disposable gloves, masks and plastic apron (and use eye protection visor/goggles if splashing is likely).
- Cover small spills (<30 mL) completely with 10 000 ppm (1%) chlorine-releasing granules (e.g. Haz-tabs, Precept, Actichlor) and wait for the fluid to absorb.
- Leave for five minutes.
- Collect granules using disposable paper towels and/or cardboard (Figure 8.11). Discard immediately as hazardous infectious clinical waste (see Chapter 10).

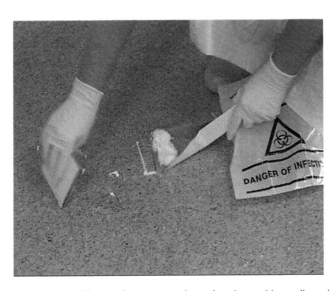

Figure 8.11 Cleaning up chlorine-releasing granules with a disposable cardboard trowel.

- Clean area with neutral, non-foaming detergent and water and dry with disposable towels.
- Dispose of towels and protective clothing as hazardous infectious clinical waste.
- Immediately wash and dry hands thoroughly.

Large spills (>30 mL)

- Use hypochlorite solution that releases 10 000 ppm (1%) chlorine.
- Wear disposable gloves, masks and plastic apron (and use eye protection visor/goggles if splashing is likely).
- If the spill is large (>30 mL), cover the area with disposable towels to limit spread and prevent aerosolization of infectious material. Wait for spill to absorb.
- Prepare chlorine-releasing solution in accordance with manufacturer's instructions.
- Carefully apply chlorine solution over the entire spillage, ensuring that paper towels are completely saturated. Leave for time recommended by the manufacturer, usually about five minutes.
- Immediately discard towels as hazardous infectious clinical waste.
- Clean area with neutral, non-foaming detergent and water, and dry area with disposable towels.
- Dispose of towels and protective clothing as hazardous infectious clinical waste.
- Wash and dry hands thoroughly.

Do remember that hypochlorite, chloramines, chlorine gas and household bleach are toxic and irritant to skin and mucous membranes via direct contact, ingestion and inhalation and should always be used with the utmost care.

REFERENCES AND WEBSITES

Bennett AM, Fulford MR, Walker JT *et al.* (2000) Microbial aerosols in general dental practice. *British Dental Journal*, **189**, 664–7.

Loveday HP, Wilson JA, Pratta RJ *et al.* (2014) Epic3: national evidence-based guidelines for preventing healthcare-associated infections in NHS Hospitals in England. *Journal of Hospital Infection*, 86(Suppl. 1), S1–S70.

Rautemaa R, Nordberg A, Wuolijoki-Saarusti K, Meurman JH. (2006) Bacterial aerosols in dental practice – a potential hospital infection problem? *Journal of Hospital Infection*, **64**, 76–81.

Chapter 9

Management of dental unit waterlines

Biofilms are complex microbial communities attached to a solid surface and embedded in an organic matrix, which makes them very resistant to removal and penetration by biocides. The biofilm with which dentists are most familiar is dental plaque and it can be appreciated that just as the relentless accumulation of dental plaque is difficult for some patients to control and remove, the control of dental unit waterline (DUWL) biofilms is a challenge for the dental profession.

Dental unit waterlines have narrow bores with a high surface area. As the water is continuously moving through the tubes of the working dental unit, how do the micro-organisms find sufficient time to form biofilms? The answer lies in the properties of fluid dynamics and geometry of dental lines (Figure 9.1). A fluid in a tube moves in layers (laminar flow). At the centre of the lumen, it travels fastest; further away from this central layer, the movement becomes slower as a result of friction. Water velocity at the tubing walls is virtually motionless, allowing bacteria to adhere and colonize the internal surface.

Microbial colonization of DUWLs results from bacteria entering by three main routes (Box 9.1). DUWLs act as 'dead legs' in the plumbing system, as water only flows through them when in use. In untreated dental units, overnight stagnation and infrequent patterns of use result in amplification of the incoming microbes to form a biofilm on the inner surface of the DUWL (Figure 9.2). Most dental units are not in active use for an average of 130 hours/week. Biofilms in DUWLs, like dental plaque, form rapidly and within a week can be shedding high bacterial counts of up to 10^{4-6} colony forming units

Basic Guide to Infection Prevention and Control in Dentistry, Second Edition.
Caroline L. Pankhurst.
© 2017 John Wiley & Sons Ltd. Published 2017 by John Wiley & Sons Ltd.
Companion website: www.wiley.com/go/pankhurst/infection-prevention

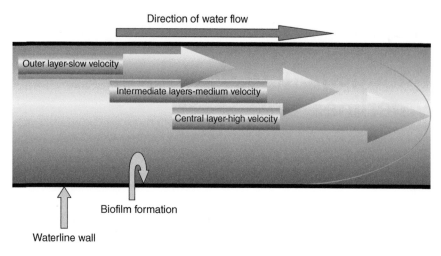

Figure 9.1 Laminar flow in a dental unit waterline.

Box 9.1   Routes of contamination of DUWLs

Low-level contamination of the incoming mains water

Retrograde movement (suck-back) of oral fluids via the dental handpiece

Contamination of the independent water reservoir systems:
* use of poor-quality water
* failure to use an aseptic technique when filling the bottle
* failure to clean the bottle adequately

(cfu)/mL into the waterline. Bacteria in biofilms are more resistant to treatment with disinfectants, ultraviolet light, metal toxicity, acid exposure and dehydration than corresponding planktonic non-attached cells.

RISK TO STAFF AND PATIENT HEALTH FROM DENTAL UNIT WATERLINES

In recent years in the USA and Europe (e.g. England 2015), 'boil water notices' have been issued in response to major incidences following water-borne contamination of the municipal water supply with *Cryptosporidium*, affecting, in some instances, thousands of consumers. Such events have fuelled public concern regarding the microbiological quality of municipal water supplies. The public's lack of confidence in water quality is illustrated by an exponential increase in sales of bottled drinking water in many countries, even though the microbiological content of many of these products vastly exceeds that found in tap water.

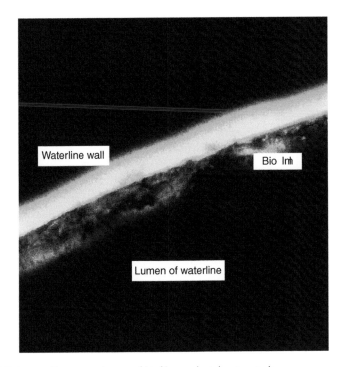

Waterline wall

Bio Inh

Lumen of waterline

Figure 9.2 Immunofluorescent image of biofilm on dental unit waterlines.

Similar concerns had been expressed over the poor quality of untreated DUWLs as bacteria present in DUWLs present both a public health and cross-infection risk. The American Dental Association Council on Scientific Affairs stated that poor microbial quality is inconsistent with patient expectations of safety in dentistry. They set a goal that water used for dental treatment should contain ≤200 cfu/mL of aerobic heterotrophic organisms, equivalent to drinking water quality. This figure is somewhat higher than the value set for potable drinking water in Europe of 100 cfu/mL of aerobic heterotrophic organisms, but is comparable with the figure given in the Department of Health's publication HTM 01-05, recommending a total viable count in the range 100–200 cfu/mL. The latter value is considered to be achievable in dental practice over the long term. Similar protocols have been adopted by other dental governing bodies around the world.

The majority of DUWL contaminants are Gram-negative aerobic environmental species, most of which are non-pathogenic and do not cause infection in immunocompetent people. However, they can impart a foul taste and odour to the water which may be detected by patients and make treatment unpleasant. Opportunistic respiratory pathogens, such as *Legionella* spp., *Pseudomonas aeruginosa* and non-tuberculosis *Mycobacterium* (NTM), are detected in a proportion of DUWLs (Table 9.1).

Table 9.1 Examples of micro-organisms isolated from DUWLs

Gram-negative bacteria	Gram-positive bacteria	Fungi	Protozoa
Legionella spp.	Lactobacillus spp.	Candida	Acanthamoeba
Pseudomonas	Actinomyces spp.	albicans	spp.
aeruginosa	Mycobacterium	Candida spp.	Giardia spp.
Acinetobacter spp.	avium	Cladosporium	Cryptosporidium
Pseudomonas spp.	Mycobacterium	spp.	spp.
Proteus vulgaris	spp.	Penicillium	Hartmannella
Fusobacterium spp.	Staphylococcus	spp.	spp.
Moraxella spp.	aureus	Phoma spp.	
Bacteroides spp.	Streptococcus	Aspergillus	
Burkholderia cepacia	spp.	spp.	
Klebsiella pneumoniae	Oral streptococci	Alternaria	
Alicaligenes		spp.	
dentrificans			

Source: Adapted from Barbot V, Robert A, Rodier M, Imbert C. (2012) Update on infectious risks associated with dental unit waterlines. *FEMS Immunol Med Microbiol*, **65**, 196–204.

Legionellae

Legionellae are distributed worldwide in all types of man-made and natural aquatic habitats. They favour warm, stagnant waters and generally occur in low numbers. Legionellae may enter the DUWL from the mains drinking water and have the ability, under suitable growth and temperature conditions, to multiply in the biofilm to reach 10^2 and 10^5 cfu/mL. By comparison, in the UK the acceptable water standards for legionellae are less than 100 legionellae in a litre of water. Typical DUWL water temperatures are between 18 and 23 °C and legionellae proliferate at temperatures between 20 and 45 °C. Hence, water in the DUWL lies within the critical growth temperature range for legionellae. Six to thirty percent of domestic hot water systems harbour legionellae and once established, they can persist for years. The reported prevalence of legionellae species in DUWLs in practices and dental schools varies widely from 0% to 68%, depending, in part, on the isolation procedures.

Legionella pneumophila serogroup 1 accounts for over 80% of *Legionella* infections. Wide variations in the recovery rates of *Legionella pneumophila* from DUWLs are observed, depending on a number of factors, including the geographic location of the dental practice or school (8% in the USA, 21.8% in Italy, 25% in London and 36% in Iran), the presence of large cold-water tanks and complex plumbing systems, thermal conditions and the brand of dental equipment. In DUWLs, legionellae are often found living symbiotically inside amoebae, protected from the action of biocides and chlorine disinfectants.

Transmission of infection occurs via inhalation of contaminated aerosol droplets or, rarely, aspiration of contaminated water by susceptible individuals.

Box 9.2 Patients at increased risk of Legionnaires' disease

- Increasing age, particularly above 50 years. Mortality is up to 30% in those over 70 years of age
- Two-thirds of patients have a co-existing illness, e.g. heart disease, diabetes, renal disease, lung disease or immunosuppression
- Smoking, particularly heavy cigarette smoking which compromises lung function
- Males are nearly three times more likely to be infected than females. Due to higher occupational exposure risk as they are more likely to be employed in outdoor occupations, construction or engineering
- Travel associated: approximately 40% of UK cases of Legionnaires' disease are due to imported cases in travellers returning from, e.g., Spain, India, China, Thailand or from cruises

---

There is no evidence of case-to-case transmission. Within the European Union, most cases occur sporadically, during the warmer summer months, and are community acquired. Legionellosis can present in three ways.

- *Legionnaires' disease* – an atypical pneumonia with a 10–30% mortality rate
- *Pontiac fever* – a mild, self-limiting, flu-like illness
- *Non-pneumonic form* – *Legionella* urinary antibodies are detected but there are no symptoms of pneumonia or Pontiac fever

Dental personnel have been shown to have higher antibody titres to *Legionella* than other non-dental control populations, suggesting occupational exposure to these potential pathogens. A dentist in the USA died from Legionnaires' disease as a result of exposure to legionellae in his surgery's DUWL. Vulnerable patients may also be susceptible to the hazards from DUWLs (see risk factors for Legionnaires' disease in Box 9.2). In a recent case report, death from Legionnaires' disease in a housebound 82-year-old Italian woman was proven conclusively to have been caused by exposure to *Legionella* growing in the DUWL and tap water at her dentist's surgery. By using molecular techniques, the authors showed that the *Legionella* strain recovered from the patient was identical to that found at her dentist's surgery. No legionellae were isolated from water samples taken at her home (Ricci *et al.*, 2012). Fortunately, overall the health risks associated with inhaling contaminated DUWL aerosols are thought to be very low in healthy individuals (Pankhurst & Coulter 2007).

Pseudomonas

Pseudomonads and related genera are the predominant bacterial genera found in DUWLs and have been isolated from up to 50% of DUWLs. Some of the species in the genera behave as opportunistic pathogens. *P. aeruginosa* accounts for 9–11% of reported nosocomial infections per annum in the USA and Europe, particularly affecting the immunocompromised, those on ventilators, burns patients and patients suffering from cystic fibrosis. The organism can thrive in low-nutrient environments such as distilled water. The latter is commonly employed by dentists as the water for DUWL reservoirs and sterilizer reservoirs. Furthermore, pseudomonads grow readily in diluted disinfectants such as chlorhexidine and iodophors and express resistance to a wide range of antibiotics. *P. aeruginosa* is a common colonizer of DUWLs and has been isolated from up to 50% of DUWLs.

There is limited direct evidence of *Pseudomonas* infection associated with exposure to a contaminated DUWL. Martin (1987) reported that *P. aeruginosa* isolated from dental abscesses in two cancer patients was identical to the *P. aeruginosa* strain recovered from the DUWLs used during their treatment. A further 78 non-compromised patients were then treated in the same *P. aeruginosa*-contaminated dental unit and were found to be transiently colonized for 3–5 weeks with the same strain of *P. aeruginosa*, but no cases of infection resulted from their exposure.

Cystic fibrosis patients are at increased risk of infection with *P. aeruginosa* from the DUWL. A recent study concluded that there was only a small risk for cystic fibrosis patients of acquiring *P. aeruginosa* from a dental treatment and the acquisition rate was comparable with the background rate of 1–2% for new infections. However, the authors caution that the accumulated risk of acquisition associated with frequent dental visits may increase the transmission rate to a clinically significant level.

Mycobacterium

Environmental mycobacteria, i.e. NTM, are widely distributed in nature and have been isolated from soil, natural water and water distribution systems, including DUWL biofilm, where they can proliferate. The colony count of NTM in DUWLs can exceed that of drinking water by a factor of 400. Thus, there is a potential risk for large numbers of NTM to be swallowed, inhaled or inoculated into oral wounds during dental treatment, leading to colonization and infection. Immunocompromised and AIDS patients are highly susceptible to opportunistic NTM. Identical strains of *Mycobacterium avium* complex have been isolated from infected AIDS patients and the drinking water tap in their homes. Fortunately, most NTM infection is asymptomatic, as studies suggest that approximately 12% of the population in the USA have been colonized by the NTM (*M. avium*) but are asymptomatic. A small number of cases of serious NTM infection have been associated directly with dental treatment and it is therefore prudent to reduce NTM contamination by effective DUWL management.

Endotoxin

Although no clinical cases of environmental bacterial infections except those due to *P. aeruginosa* have been directly associated with dental procedures, the bacterial cell wall of Gram-negative bacteria is a potent source of endotoxin. Endotoxin can cause localized inflammation, fever and shock. A high bacterial load in the DUWL usually equates with a high endotoxin concentration. A consequence of inhaled endotoxin exposure is the triggering or exacerbation of asthma. Data from a large practice-based cross-sectional study reported a temporal association between occupational exposure to contaminated DUWLs with aerobic counts of >200 cfu/mL and development of occupational asthma in the subgroup of dentists in whom asthma arose following the commencement of dental training (Pankhurst *et al.*, 2005). The US Pharmacopeia sets a limit for endotoxin for irrigation sterile water of 0.25 endotoxin units/mL. Endotoxin has been detected in dental water up to 500–2560 units/mL.

METHODS TO REDUCE THE BIOFILM

Dental unit waterline management regulations and guidelines and commercially available decontamination systems are specifically designed to reduce and maintain environmental Gram-negative aerobic bacteria and oral bacteria at an acceptable level ($\leq$200 cfu/mL) in the water issuing from the DUWL.

The rationale behind the regulations is to:

- overcome the resistance mechanism operating within the biofilm
- prevent the survival and amplification of pathogens, e.g. legionellae
- prevent recolonization of the tubing once the biofilm is removed
- counteract the effects of low-volume intermittent use that leads to stagnation of the entire water column within DUWLs for extended periods during the day
- prevent overnight and weekend water stagnation.

The overall aim is to ensure that there are a safe number of planktonic microbes in the irrigation water when it reached the mouth or is aerosolized, i.e. less than 200 cfu/mL. As there are multiple entry points for microbes into DUWLs, no single method is completely effective and a combination of control measure is usually required, as outlined in Box 9.3.

Dental units should be drained down and waterlines disinfected twice daily.

> ## Box 9.3 Key recommendations to maintain the quality of DUWLs
>
> - All waterlines and airlines should be fitted with antiretraction valves
> - An independent reservoir bottled water system should be used to supply the dental waterlines
> - Fill reservoir bottles with fresh distilled or reverse osmosis water in preference to potable mains water
> - Biocides should be used in the reservoir bottle and waterlines (applied according to manufacturer's instructions)
> - Dental unit waterlines, reservoir bottles and pipework should be drained down, flushed and disinfected with biocide according to manufacturer's instructions twice daily, e.g. beginning and end of the day
> - At the end of the day, reservoir bottles should be disinfected with biocide, rinsed with fresh reverse osmosis or distilled water, drained and stored dry and inverted overnight
> - Dental unit waterlines should be flushed at the beginning and end of the day for two minutes and for 20–30 seconds between patients
> - If point-of-use antimicrobial filters are fitted in the line, they should be replaced daily or according to manufacturer's instructions
> - Infrequently used DUWLs should be flushed on a regular basis (at least weekly)
> - A separate sterile water delivery system or saline should be used for invasive surgical procedures
> - Regulations for a physical air gap on dental equipment should be followed to prevent back-siphonage
>
> Source: Summarized from guidance published in HTM 01-05 and HSG 274.

Value and limitations of flushing

Flushing reduces the bacterial count by approximately 97%, but will not reduce the total count to ≤ 200 cfu/mL; nor will it remove the biofilm. So, in most units flushing is insufficient on its own to control the bacterial count in the DUWL. Flushing at the beginning of the day for two minutes removes any residual biocide in addition to biofilm dislodged by biocide treatment regimes. Care should be taken by the operator to avoid splatter and aerosol exposure during DUWL flushing and masks and eyewear should be donned.

Flushing the waterlines between patients for 20–30 seconds helps to prevent cross-contamination by removing oral fluids. These are introduced into the DUWL via suck-back through the handpieces, which is caused by the negative pressure generated in the handpiece when the foot pedal is released. An estimated 1 mL of microbe-laden oral fluid can be aspirated into the DUWL if antiretraction valves have not been fitted. Antiretraction valves require regular maintenance otherwise they act as a scaffold for bacterial growth and become clogged and cease to function. Flushing also has the advantage of drawing up fresh biocide into the DUWL and thereby facilitating disinfection of the line.

It is important to prevent the development of the biofilm as it is difficult to remove once established. Check valves are fitted to the waterline to reduce gross contamination.

Biocides

Thermal controls are the ideal method to control the growth of legionellae but are not suitable for dental unit waterlines. A vast range of chemical and non-chemical products have been developed for the maintenance of dental unit waterlines, includingcontinuous and intermittent biocides, point-of-use microbial filters, electrochemically activated water, junction box UV treatment, etc. National guidelines recommend the use of biocides to control biofilm formation. The biocide can be introduced with a pressurized pump system or via an independent reservoir bottled water system. Some dental units are fitted with an automated continuous biocide dosing system.

Box 9.4 gives examples of the types of biocides that are appropriate for use in dental unit waterlines. Note that continuous dosing products are imbibed and inhaled by the patient. Therefore, they contain lower concentrations of disinfectant to prevent toxicity to the oral and respiratory tissues and must be able to be tolerated by the patient. Their efficacy is dependent on their continuous presence in the waterlines. Intermittent biocides are

---

Box 9.4   Biocides and treatments used in the disinfection of DUWLs (examples only – the list is not exhaustive)

- Hydrogen peroxide
- Hydrogen peroxide and silver ions
- Alkaline peroxide
- Citric acid formulation
- Chlorhexidine gluconate formulation
- Electrochemically activated water
- Peracetic acid
- Tetrasodium EDTA
- Quaternary ammonium formulations
- Chlorine dioxide
- Povidine iodine cartridges
- Ultraviolet

See also Table A.3 in the Appendix.

---

formulated at a higher concentration as they are only used as a purge for short durations. Tissue toxicity is less of a problem as they do not come into direct patient contact. After purging, the lines are then rinsed thoroughly with fresh (less than 12 hours old) reverse osmosis or distilled water so that the patient is not exposed to any residual disinfectant. A large multicentre European study found that the peroxide-based products were particularly effective when evaluated over long-term use. Continuous dosing regimens for disinfecting the DUWLs performed better than once-daily intermittent applications of biocide (Schel *et al.*, 2006). Not all products remove the biofilm completely, so regular dosing according to the manufacturer's instructions is required to control the bacterial count. Hence, the most recent guidelines recommend that intermittent products are used to purge the waterlines twice daily to prevent regrowth of the biofilm, as biofilms can reform in approximately eight hours.

Only use a biocide that is recommended as compatible with your particular dental unit as unsuitable products can damage internal components resulting in leaks or blockages (O'Donnell *et al.*, 2011). Hypochlorite is an effective biocide and is used widely to maintain swimming pools. However, its use in DUWLs is limited by the corrosive effects it has on metals (e.g. handpieces) and the unwanted release of mercury from amalgam. Therefore, it has been superseded by non-corrosive biocide products, specifically designed for DUWLs. Hypochlorite use is mainly confined to 'shock treatment' in situations where the waterlines and water distribution system are known to be contaminated with legionellae (Ricci *et al.*, 2012).

Alternative measures to biocides

Disposable microbial filters placed in line as close as possible to the handpiece will prevent suspended bacteria entering the handpiece, but do not remove the biofilm. If used according to the manufacturer's instructions, these devices can produce DUWL water of drinking water standard or better.

Water purification systems treat the water coming into the dental unit. They kill or remove micro-organisms by methods such as filtration, electrochemically activated water or ultraviolet light. One advantage of these methods is that they may delay biofilm formation on water lines or synergize with other treatment measures. As they are not discharged in the effluent water, they are non-polluting to the environment and are less likely to select for antimicrobial-resistant species than biocides used in DUWLs.

> Fill bottles with fresh distilled or reverse osmosis water in preference to potable mains water.

Type of water used to supply the DUWL

Independent reservoir bottled water systems are either an integral part of the dental chair or can be installed separately (Figure 9.3). The main advantage is that they draw fluids from the reservoir bottle filled with reverse osmosis or distilled water, or alternatively a dilute biocide in an aqueous solution, and bypass the municipal water supply, thus avoiding contamination of the DUWL with legionellae, NTM and other water-borne respiratory pathogens. However, such systems alone cannot reliably improve the quality of the treatment water, as biofilms are able to form within the bottle unless carefully managed. Regular disinfection of the inside of the bottle and flushing of the waterlines with a biocide are required to reduce adherent microbial biofilms.

> Prevent contamination of the mains water supply using a physical air gap.

Prevention of back-siphonage into the mains

European Union regulations state that there should be a physical gap or type A air gap separating the DUWL from the mains water supply in order to prevent back-siphonage of clinical material into the municipal supply. Compliance can be achieved either by installing a storage tank fitted with water piping with a regulation air gap or by an independent bottled water system to supply water directly to the DUWLs and handpieces.

> Use sterile water for implant, periodontal and oral surgery irrigation.

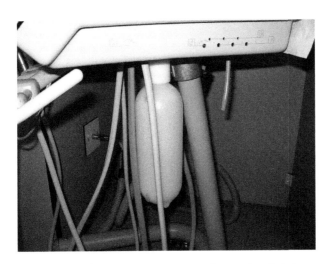

Figure 9.3 Independent bottled water system integrated into a dental chair.

Irrigation water for invasive procedures

Sterile water delivered in a separate delivery system is required for minor oral surgery (MOS) procedures, periodontal and implant surgery (Figure 9.4). The use of terile or distilled water *per se* is of no help in solving this problem if it is used within dental lines already contaminated with a biofilm. For MOS, implant and periodontal surgery and other invasive procedures, the guidance in the UK and from the ADA (American Dental Association) is to irrigate with sterile water or saline. Importantly, for these sterile solutions to remain uncontaminated, they need to be delivered through devices other than the DUWL. A variety of delivery systems are commercially available incorporating pump and bagged sterile solutions or fully autoclavable assemblies of reservoirs and handpiece tubing to be used with sterile water (see Figure 9.4). The disadvantage of these systems is that they can be expensive to purchase and more cumbersome and often less convenient to use than conventional delivery systems. However, when small volumes are required, a sterile disposable syringe filled with saline is a suitable alternative.

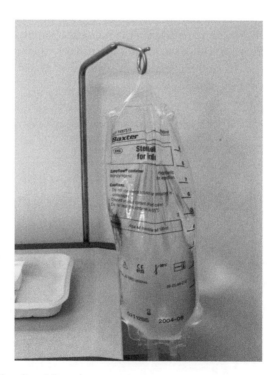

Figure 9.4 Sterile saline delivery bag.

Box 9.5   Thermal control of legionellae in the dental water system

Hot-water plumbing
- Avoid storage of water between 20 and 45 °C
- Hot water should be stored at ≥60 °C
- Aim is to achieve a hot water temperature of 55 °C at all points of use within one minute of turning on the hot tap
- Maintain cleanliness of system, e.g. reduce scale and deposits
- Use a thermostatic mixer tap for hand basins set at 38–44 °C to avoid scalding. Recommended to use hazard notice stating, 'Be careful, very hot water'
- Flush infrequently used taps for several minutes on a weekly basis to reduce risks associated with stagnation and low water usage

Cold-water plumbing
- Site cold-water tanks in a cool place with thermal insulation
- Aim is to achieve cold water temperature of below 20 °C after running the taps for two minutes
- Introduce measures to reduce stagnation (e.g. remove or shorten length of dead leg pipes, remove redundant taps)
- In hard water areas, softening of the cold water supply to the hot water distribution system should be considered to reduce the risk of scale being deposited at the base of the calorifier and heating coils
- Keep the amount of water stored to a minimum, i.e. equivalent to no more 12 hours' usage

Monitoring and recording
- Temperature of sentinel outlets to hot and cold taps; inlets to sentinel thermal mixer valves; water leaving and returning to calorifier should be checked monthly
- Biannual monitoring should be done to ensure that the incoming cold water to the premises is below 20 °C at the ball valve outlet of the cold-water storage tank
- Water engineer should inspect and maintain the cleanliness of the system on an annual basis, e.g. inspect tanks and water heaters for sludge and debris, clean and remove if necessary
- If foul taste and/or foul odour problems are noted then a microbiological investigation may be required as this could signal development of conditions that could promote growth of legionellae. Water samples for analysis should be sent to an accredited laboratory; dip slides are not recommended for legionellae detection as they can give false-negative results

Source: Based on legislation and guidance in Health & Safety Executive (2013)
Legionnaires' disease: The control of legionella bacteria in water systems. Approved Code of Practice L8, 4th edn, HTM 01-05 and HSG 274.

CONTROL OF LEGIONELLAE IN THE DENTAL PRACTICE WATER SUPPLY

In the dental practice, there are other sources of water besides the DUWL that the dentist has to control to prevent legionellae contamination, namely the hot and cold water supply to the sinks, plumbed equipment and toilets, all of which if contaminated could potentially have health consequences for the public. Therefore, there is a legal requirement for dentists to control the legionellae bacteria in all their water systems.

In order to comply with their legal duties, dentists, with the help of a Competent Person (Water Engineer), should identify and assess the potential risks for legionellae proliferation and aerosolization within the dental surgery plumbing. Unlike in dental waterlines, legionellae in the water system can be effectively controlled with thermal measures that avoid the storage of water between 20 and 45 °C, the preferred growth temperature range for legionellae. The Competent Person on behalf of the dental practice must prepare a written control scheme (water plan) for preventing and controlling the risk from legionellae in practice water systems and DUWLs. The Water Engineer should maintain the cleanliness of the hot and cold plumbing system and boiler and train the dental team in where and how to take sentinel water temperatures. An annual inspection, cleaning and testing of the water system by the engineer is recommended.

The dental practice has a duty to record and monitor the water temperatures in the hot and cold water systems on a monthly, six-monthly and annual basis as set out in the water plan. Records must be retained for five years. A brief summary of the key advice in the legislation and guidelines pertaining to dental practices is outlined in Box 9.5. For a full explanation of the guidelines, please consult the Approved Code of Practice 'Legionnaire's disease: The control of legionella bacteria in water systems', HSG 274 and HTM 01-05.

REFERENCES AND WEBSITES

Health & Safety Executive (2013) Legionnaires' disease: The control of legionella bacteria in water systems. Approved Code of Practice L8, 4th edn. Available at: www.hse.gov.uk/ (accessed 4 November 2016).

Health & Safety Executive (2013) Legionnaires' disease: Technical guidance. Part 3: The control of legionella bacteria in other risk systems. HSG 274, Part 3. Available at: www.hse.gov.uk/pubns/books/hsg274.htm (accessed 4 November 2016).

Martin MV. (1987)The significance of the bacterial contamination of dental unit water systems. *British Dental Journal*, **163**, 152–154.

O'Donnell MJ, Boyle M, Swan J, Russell RJ, Coleman DC. (2011) Management of dental unit waterline biofilms in the 21th century. *Future Microbiology*, **6**, 1209–1226.

Pankhurst CL, Coulter WA. (2007) Do contaminated dental unit waterlines pose a risk of infection? *Journal of Dentistry*, **35**, 712–720.

Pankhurst CL, Coulter WA, Philpott-Howard JJ *et al.* (2005) Evaluation of potential risk of occupational asthma in dentist exposed to contaminated dental unit water lines. *Primary Dental Care*, **12**, 53–59.

Ricci ML, Fontana S, Pinci F *et al.* (2012) Pneumonia associated with a dental unit waterline. *Lancet*, **379**, 684.

Schel AJ, Marsh PD, Bradshaw DJ *et al.* (2006) Comparison of the efficacies of disinfectants to control microbial contamination in dental unit water systems in general dental practices across the European Union. *Applied Environmental Microbiology*, **73**, 1380–1387.

Chapter 10

Healthcare waste management

LEGISLATION ON HAZARDOUS WASTE DISPOSAL

The healthcare sector is a major producer of waste. According to the WHO, worldwide about 15% of the total waste generated by healthcare activities is hazardous material that may be infectious, toxic or radioactive. Infectious healthcare waste contains potentially harmful micro-organisms, which is a hazard to anyone who has contact with it until it is made safe. Clinical wastes from healthcare facilities can act as a reservoir of antibiotic-resistant organisms, which if not managed correctly can contaminate the environment, affecting both soil and water supplies. In those areas of the world with poor sanitation, this could lead to the transmission of drug-resistant microbes to the surrounding population, as occurred with the multidrug-resistant strain New Delhi metallo-β-lactamase (NDM)-producing Enterobacteriaceae.

Healthcare waste in the form of disinfectants, cytotoxic pharmaceuticals, antibiotics or other byproducts released during incineration, such as mercury, may also poison and pollute the natural environment. Effluent waste antibiotics are environmentally persistent and are a particular problem as they select for resistance genes in environmental water and soil bacteria. In turn, the resistance genes can be shared with bacteria normally found in foods for human consumption, as well as in wildlife, thus completing the circle in the chain of transmission by providing a route whereby the antibiotic resistance genes are transmitted to human pathogens on the hands or in the gut.

Basic Guide to Infection Prevention and Control in Dentistry, Second Edition.
Caroline L. Pankhurst.
© 2017 John Wiley & Sons Ltd. Published 2017 by John Wiley & Sons Ltd.
Companion website: www.wiley.com/go/pankhurst/infection-prevention

One of the primary goals in waste management strategies across the UK and European Union is to manage waste safely and sustainably by:

- reducing the volume of waste produced per capita
- limiting the number of landfill sites
- protecting the environment from pollution by hazardous effluents.

This 'green' approach to healthcare waste is reflected in national legislation, namely the Environmental Protection Act 1990 and Hazardous Waste Regulations 2005 (Special Waste Regulations in Scotland). The registered manager and the dental practice under the legislation are defined as a waste 'producer'. They have full responsibility and a duty of care for ensuring that their waste is properly managed, recovered or disposed of safely, according to national and international guidelines. Waste must only be transferred to an authorized waste contractor. As some healthcare wastes may prove hazardous to people who are exposed to them, they are subject to stringent controls and are referred to as 'controlled wastes'. As an employer, the dentist is responsible for protecting all members of their dental team, patients, the general public and waste disposal contractors from accidental exposure to hazardous waste produced by activities at their dental practice. All members of the dental team can make a contribution to protecting the environment by reducing the amount of unnecessary waste produced and recycling or recovering waste (e.g. metals) whenever possible.

On a practical level, each dental practice is required to prepare its own waste policy and to identify which member(s) of staff are responsible for overseeing the local management of healthcare waste, including:

- correctly segregating hazardous from non-hazardous waste
- ensuring that waste is stored safely and securely on the dental premises
- packaging waste appropriately for transport
- describing waste accurately on documentation that accompanies the waste to an authorized waste site
- retaining records and returns on waste management
- undertaking a waste audit every two years
- training staff so that they are aware of the waste procedures.

Fortunately, in the UK, the dentist is guided through this complex web of national and international waste legislation by a best practice guide entitled 'Environment and Sustainability HTM 07-01: Safe Management of Healthcare Waste'. Variations exist in the interpretation of the legislation in the devolved countries of the UK and readers can view these via the hyperlink on the companion website www.wiley.com/go/pankhurst/infection-prevention. In Scotland, the term 'hazardous' waste is replaced with the term 'special waste' but for simplification, the term 'hazardous waste' will be used throughout this chapter. The key features of HTM 07-01 are outlined in Box 10.1.

Box 10.1   Key features from HTM 07-01 on premises notification and disposal of healthcare waste

- Dentists as producers of healthcare waste have a duty of care to ensure that all healthcare waste is managed and disposed of properly.
- It is a statutory requirement in England and Wales for waste producers to segregate hazardous and non-hazardous waste at source since it is not permissible to dispose of hazardous and non-hazardous material at the same landfill site.
- Transfer and consignment notes must contain a written description of the waste and the appropriate European Waste Catalogue (EWC) codes.
- Dental practices (consignors) in England and Wales (not Scotland or Northern Ireland) of hazardous waste must notify their premises to the Environment Agency annually.* A dental premise is exempted from notification if it produces less than 500 kg of hazardous waste material per year (which includes hazardous non-clinical items such as fridges, TVs, computer screens) and the hazardous waste is removed from the premises by a registered carrier.
- Movement of hazardous waste from premises that are not either notified (registered) or exempted is prohibited; in doing so a criminal offence is committed.
- Each dental premise producing waste is assigned a unique six-digit premise reference code that is used to identify and track the movement of the waste.
- Owners of multiple practices are required to register each practice separately.
- The producer must ensure that the waste falls within the terms of the waste contractor's waste management licence, permit or exemption for the final disposal of the waste.
- The producer must keep transfer notes from the waste carrier for two years and consignment notes and returns from waste disposal contractor for three years.

Modified from 'Environment and Sustainability HTM 07-01: Safe Management of Healthcare Waste – 2013'.

* In Northern Ireland and Scotland, the waste producer must prenotify either NIEA or SEPA respectively, prior to each collection and movement of hazardous waste.

TYPES OF WASTE

Dental practices generate both hazardous and non-hazardous healthcare waste that can be categorized into seven waste streams (Figure 10.1).

The remainder of this chapter will focus on the disposal of waste generated by dental treatment. For information on the disposal or recycling of electronic and domestic waste, please refer to the Department for Environment, Food, and Rural Affairs and Environment Agency websites listed on the companion website www.wiley.com/go/pankhurst/infection-prevention.

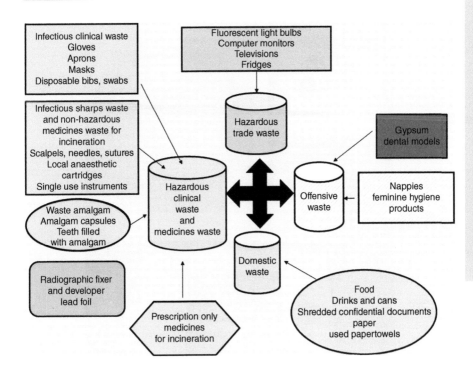

Figure 10.1 Dental waste streams

Hazardous waste streams

1. Infectious clinical waste
2. Amalgam waste
3. Radiographic waste
4. Electrical and electronic wastes

Non-hazardous waste streams

5. Medicines waste
6. 'Offensive waste' and gypsum
7. Domestic waste.

WHAT IS HAZARDOUS WASTE?

Not all clinical waste is hazardous waste.

Clinical waste generated by healthcare activities includes a broad range of materials, from used needles and syringes to soiled swabs and dressings, body parts, diagnostic samples, blood, amalgam, chemicals, pharmaceuticals,

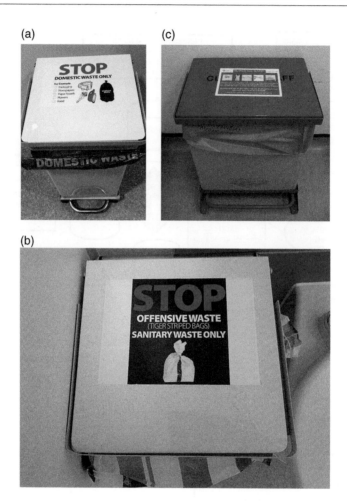

Figure 10.2 Types of waste sacks used for segregating domestic, offensive and infectious waste. (a) Clear waste sack for domestic waste. (b) Black and yellow striped waste sack for Sanpro offensive waste. (c) Orange waste sack in a leak-proof, flame-retardant, foot-operated pedal bin.

medical devices and radioactive materials. Waste has to be segregated as not all healthcare waste is hazardous so that it can be treated appropriately to make it safe (Figure 10.2, Box 10.2).

For a waste to be defined as hazardous, it must have one or more properties that are hazardous to health or the environment:

• explosive, oxidizing, highly flammable, flammable, irritant, infectious, toxic, carcinogenic, teratogenic, mutagenic, harmful, releases toxic gases, sensitizing, ecotoxic.

Prior to disposal in landfill sites, the traditional method for reducing the volume and mass of clinical waste and making it safe has been incineration. But a

Box 10.2 EWC codes for use in dental practice

Chapters 9 and 15 of EWC
- 09 01 01* X-ray photographic developer
- 09 01 04* X-ray photographic fixer
- 09 01 07 X-ray film
- 15 01 04 X-ray lead foils from dentistry

Chapter 18 of EWC
Waste from natal care, diagnosis, treatment or prevention of diseases in humans
- 18 01 01 Sharps except 18 01 03*
- 18 01 02 Body parts and organs including blood bags and blood preserves (except 18 01 03*)
- 18 01 03* Waste whose collection and disposal is subject to special requirements in order to prevent infection
- 18 01 04 Waste whose collection and disposal is not subject to special requirements in order to prevent infection, e.g. dressings, plaster casts, linen, disposable clothing
- 18 01 06* Chemicals consisting of dangerous substances
- 18 01 07 Chemicals other than those listed in 18 01 06*
- 18 01 08* Cytotoxic and cytostatic medicines
- 18 01 09 Medicines other than those mentioned in 18 01 08*
- 18 01 10* Amalgam waste from dental care

* Refers to hazardous waste regardless of threshold concentration.

burgeoning body of evidence has questioned the efficacy and safety of incineration. Of particular concern is chemical and biological pollution from exhaust emissions, especially when incinerators are located in residential or environmentally sensitive areas. For instance, incineration of heavy metals or materials with high metal content (in particular lead, mercury and cadmium) can lead to the spread of toxic metals in the environment, which is why these substances are segregated into separate waste streams. Temperature gradients form in the incinerator exhaust stack, allowing pathogenic bacteria to survive in the cooler zones at the base of the stack. Viable bacteria can be released from exhaust flues under certain circumstances. Incinerated materials containing chlorine can generate dioxins and furans, which are human carcinogens and have been associated with a range of adverse health effects. However, state-of-the-art incinerators operating at 850–1100 °C that are fitted with specific gas-cleaning equipment are able to comply with the international emission standards for dioxins and furans.

These and similar concerns have prompted the introduction of more reliable and environment-friendly methods that produce a lower carbon footprint. These technologies, which employ heat in the form of autoclaving, microwaving or

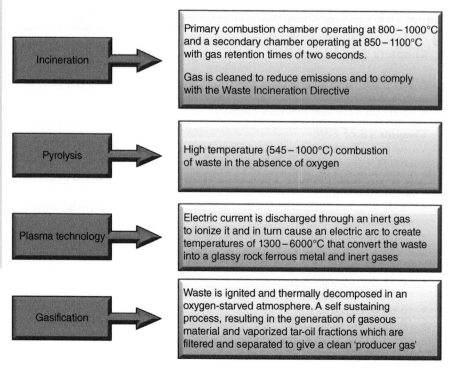

Figure 10.3 High-temperature processes.

chemical treatments, are referred to collectively as 'alternative technology methods'. Heat processes can be divided into high- and low-temperature methods (Figures 10.3 and 10.4). All of these processes are intended to render the waste non-hazardous, unrecognizable and acceptable for landfill. In general, alternative technology methods operate at lower temperatures than those generated during incineration. Industrial microwaving, for example, exposes the waste to temperatures in the range of 95–98 °C but low temperatures are unsuitable for wastes containing metal objects, body parts, toxic chemicals and radioactive substances.

It is essential that the waste disposal contractor is made aware of the exact composition of the waste so that it can be treated using the most appropriate process. Hence, the emphasis on correctly labelling waste containers, as well as on accurate completion of the accompanying waste documentation. Dental practices are also required by the legislation to complete a waste audit to confirm that all their waste is entering the correct waste streams and is disposed of into appropriate waste containers (Table 10.1). Personal protective equipment comprises the bulk of the clinical waste produced in dentistry and this can be effectively treated with alternative technology processes. Incineration is reserved for sharps, medicines and anatomical wastes. Once a waste is rendered free of infection using either low-temperature technologies or incineration, then it is no longer considered to be hazardous and can go to landfill.

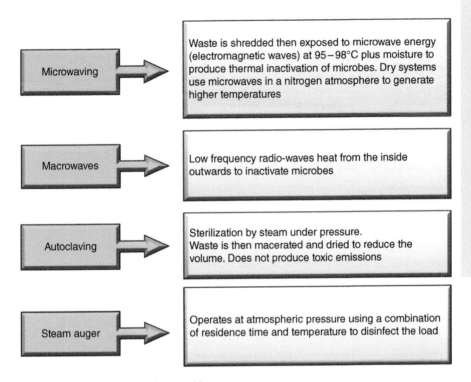

Figure 10.4 Alternative non-burn and low-temperature processes.

CLINICAL WASTE SEGREGATION AND CLASSIFICATION

> All waste must be segregated according to its European Waste Catalogue code.

The dentist has a statutory duty to segregate waste into different waste streams and consign the waste correctly, i.e. label waste for collection with a brief written description of the waste and the appropriate European Waste Catalogue (EWC) code. Developed by the European Commission and applicable across all the states of the European Union, the EWC code classifies individual waste products under 20 main chapter headings that are associated with an industrial sector. Each type of waste product is assigned a six-digit code; the final two digits are unique to the waste. Hazardous waste is marked with an asterisk (*) after the code number. The chapters applicable to dental healthcare waste are Chapter 18 of the EWC for the waste from natal care, diagnosis, treatment or prevention of diseases in humans (see Box 10.2) and Chapters 9 and 15 of the EWC for the consignment of X-ray fixer and developer and lead foil, which is applicable to those dental practices that are not using digital radiographic systems.

Table 10.1 Colour code denotes identification, segregation and method of waste disposal

Colour code	Type of waste	Mode of treatment and disposal
Black or clear waste sacks	Domestic – non-hazardous trade waste, e.g. paper/magazines, food packaging	Landfill or recycling (20 03 01)
Orange waste sacks	Clinical waste – infectious: PPE, swabs, dressings, disposable suction tips, plastic sleeves/cling film contaminated with blood/saliva	Alternative treatment plant or incineration (18 01 03*)
Yellow-lidded waste disposal containers	Clinical waste – mixed sharps and pharmaceutical waste, e.g. syringe, needles, sutures, used drug vials, partially or fully discharged local anaesthetic cartridges, teeth not filled with amalgam	Incineration (18 01 03* & 18 01 09)
Yellow and black striped waste sacks	Non-infectious 'offensive waste stream', e.g. nappies, feminine hygiene products, Sanpro Uncontaminated personal protective equipment, e.g. no body fluids, amalgam or chemicals	Must be suitably packaged but does not require any treatment prior to deep landfill (18 01 04)
White-lidded receptacles	Dental amalgam and mercury: non-infectious: dental mercury and amalgam waste, amalgam capsules and excess, contents of amalgam separator Dental amalgam infectious clinical waste: teeth filled with amalgam	Recovery of mercury & metals (18 01 10*)
Blue-lidded rigid waste disposal containers	Clinical waste: non-cytotoxic and cytostatic medicines, e.g. expired emergency drugs, painkillers, antibiotics	Incineration (18 01 09)
Gypsum waste sacks	Plaster cast waste: gypsum or calcium sulphate study or working models	Gypsum recovery or landfill in a separate dedicated area for gypsum (18 01 04)
Red-lidded waste disposal containers	**In Scotland**, a special waste stream is used for individual potentially toxic products, e.g. dental radiography chemicals, amalgam and amalgam-filled teeth	Specialized disposal

Classification of infectious clinical waste

Infectious clinical waste is defined as:

> Substances containing viable micro-organisms or their toxins which are known or reliably believed to cause disease in man or other living organisms.

Note that even organisms or toxins causing minor infections, such as dental caries or periodontal disease, are included within the definition of infectious waste. On behalf of the dental profession, the regulatory authority has decided to interpret the definition of infectious waste in line with Standard Precautions for Infection Control (see Chapter 2), whereby all clinical waste contaminated with traces of body fluids such as saliva or blood is to be consigned as infectious hazardous waste and labelled as 18 01 03, for example used gloves, masks, plastic aprons, needles sutures, scalpels, etc. Occasionally, PPE is worn but is not exposed to body fluids from splatter and this can be disposed of as non-hazardous waste 18 01 04. Excluded from the definition of hazardous waste are items such as disposable paper towels used for drying washed hands, which as the hands are clean after hand hygiene are considered as non-hazardous and can be segregated for recycling with other paper waste.

Classification of anatomical waste and teeth

Recognizable body parts (e.g. surgical or pathological specimens) are considered to be offensive to the general public and must be disposed of into yellow-lidded waste receptacles for incineration that reduces them to ash. Teeth, although body parts, are not considered likely to cause offence if they are accidently discovered in treated waste and therefore do not need to be incinerated. Patients should be offered the option to keep their extracted tooth, a popular choice with children hoping for a visit from the 'tooth fairy' who will exchange their tooth for a gift. Unwanted extracted teeth are disposed of as infectious sharps waste (18 01 03). Amalgam-containing teeth must never be incinerated or disposed of using alternative technology methods as toxic mercury compounds are released into the atmosphere by these processes. Instead, they should be segregated from other healthcare waste. Teeth should be stored in a white-lidded rigid container containing a mercury suppressant prior to appropriate recovery/disposal of the amalgam by a licensed specialist waste disposal contractor.

The patient or the dentist may wish to donate the tooth to a dental school for training or research. In the UK (except Scotland), under the Human Tissue Act written consent must be obtained from the patient before the tooth can be passed onto a dental school or other third party licensed with the Human Tissue Authority. Before sending them on, teeth should be disinfected if filled with amalgam or steam sterilized if amalgam free. Unwanted teeth can be used within the dental practice for education, in-house training or clinical audit and quality assurance without the requirement for written consent from the patient.

Never incinerate amalgam waste because it releases toxic mercury compounds.

Classification of gypsum waste

Study models or working models made of plaster contain gypsum. If models are disposed of in domestic landfill sites and mixed with food waste, the bacteria in the food break down the gypsum to release hydrogen sulphide gas, a common cause of 'acid rain'. This is a toxic pollutant of soils, waters and forests that is harmful to trees, fish and other aquatic animals. For this reason, gypsum is prohibited from domestic landfill sites. Models should be segregated from other waste, coded as 18 01 04, and either sent for recycling as gypsum or for disposal in a specifically designated landfill site. In a small number of cases, the model may become contaminated with body fluids if the appliance or crown is retried on the model after insertion in the patient's mouth. In this case models should then be disposed of in an orange waste sack as an infectious waste.

Classification of prescription-only medicines waste

Prescription-only medicines (POM) fall into three categories.

1. Cytotoxic and cytostatic medicines (i.e. kills or inhibits human cells),which are not usually used or disposed of during routine dental treatment.
2. Pharmaceutically active but not cytotoxic and cytostatic (e.g. local anaesthetic solution, emergency drugs, painkillers, antibiotics).
3. Not pharmaceutically active and possessing no hazardous properties. Examples include saline (e.g. used as an irrigant) and glucose.

Only cytotoxic or cytostatic medicines possessing hazardous characteristics – toxic, carcinogenic, teratogenic or mutagenic – are classified as hazardous waste. Classification of a drug as a POM may change over time and can vary from country to country. For the latest classification, consult published national pharmacopoeia such as the British National Formulary or publications produced by organizations such as the Food and Drug Administration in the USA.

The definition of medicinal waste is broad; it includes:

- expired, unused, spilt, contaminated pharmaceutical products, drugs, vaccines and sera
- disposable items used in the handling of pharmaceuticals, such as packaging contaminated with drug residues, gloves, masks, connecting tubing, syringes and drug vials
- fully or partially discharged local anaesthetic cartridges.

However, regardless of its classification, the disposal route for all POM waste is incineration at a suitably authorized facility. Only the high temperatures generated during incineration can sufficiently degrade POMs to render them safe and non-polluting to the natural environment. Microwaving and other low-temperature technologies are inadequate for this task.

A dental practice can return unused or expired medicines to a local pharmacy. Please note that the same legal requirements and duty of care apply as when transferring them to a waste contractor. A waste transfer note should be completed, signed and retained for two years by both the pharmacy and the dental practice.

Classification of radiographic materials

Radiographic fixer and developer solutions are classified as hazardous. These hazardous wastes should be stored in a leak-proof, rigid container prior to collection by a suitably licensed waste contractor for either recovery or disposal. Silver is recovered from X-ray film and lead from lead foil from radiograph packets during waste disposal (see Box 10.2).

AMALGAM WASTE AND INSTALLATION OF AMALGAM SEPARATORS

> Amalgam waste must be removed using an amalgam separator and disposed of as a hazardous waste.

Dental amalgam is classified as a hazardous waste with its own EWC code (18 01 10). In practical terms, this means that the surgery must segregate all forms of waste amalgam or mercury from other waste streams. Amalgam released during the removal of old restorations must be prevented from entering the practice's effluent water pipes via the spittoon and suction hoses. Discharging of hazardous waste including amalgam into the sewers is not permitted in most countries, including amongst others the UK, European Union, USA and Australia.

MERCURY IN THE ENVIRONMENT

Dentistry's contribution to the levels of mercury in the natural environment is negligible. Nevertheless, dentists are obliged to do all they can to protect the environment from mercury. Amalgamation of mercury for dental restorations produces a stable compound that does not readily convert to methyl mercury, the form that enters the food chain with detrimental, toxic consequences to aquatic mammals, fish and other species and ultimately to human health. Any clinical waste contaminated with amalgam or amalgam capsules must never be disposed of with other types of clinical waste or poured down the sink. Solid amalgam waste awaiting collection should be stored in white-lidded rigid containers under a mercury suppressant. Amalgam aspirated from the mouth is removed by an amalgam separator fitted in the waste line of the suction apparatus to stop amalgam entering the drains (effluent water system) or sewers.

Fitting of amalgam separators

Chair-side traps and vacuum filters are adequate for trapping large particles of debris, but are not fine enough to remove small suspensions of mercury particles. Hence, simple filters and gauzes were superseded by amalgam separators that meet the BS EN ISO 11143:2000 standard. Amalgam separators operate by employing one or more of the following technologies: sedimentation, fine filtration, centrifugal force and ion exchange. Separators can be retrofitted to existing dental unit suction equipment or alternatively fitted to a central suction unit serving multiple surgeries. If all the waste pipes carrying waste amalgam discharge from individual surgeries via the same effluent water pipeline, then a separator can be installed on the ultimate outflow pipe from the premises. Safe removal of the waste mercury and disposal of the separated material is the final stage of the process. The dentist is responsible for ensuring that the mercury waste is collected and treated by a waste contractor whose facilities are licensed for the recovery and disposal of hazardous amalgam waste.

Never use a vacuum cleaner or suction apparatus to clear up a mercury/amalgam spillage as this will vaporize the mercury, causing toxic fumes to be vented into the surgery. A mercury spillage kit (Box 10.3) should be kept readily available for use in the event of an accident.

Box 10.3　Mercury spillage kit

- Bulb aspirator for the collection of large drops of mercury
- White-lidded leak proof receptacle fitted with a seal and mercury suppressant (absorbent paste made of equal parts of calcium hydroxide, flowers of sulphur and water)
- Vapour mask
- Disposable gloves
- Paper towels
- Conduct a risk assessment for mercury spillages, draw up a local policy for handling spillages and train staff accordingly

DISPOSAL AND HANDLING OF HAZARDOUS WASTE IN THE SURGERY

Good practice guide: handling of hazardous waste sacks

- Segregate waste according to the waste streams shown in Box 10.2 and Table 10.1.
- Best practice recommendation is to use nationally accepted colour-coded waste sacks to distinguish between different types of waste streams (see Table 10.1).
- Never use waste sacks to dispose of sharps (i.e. any item that could potentially puncture the bag) or liquids; these should be disposed of in puncture- and leak-proof receptacles (bins).
- Use appropriately labelled UN-type leak- and tear-resistant orange waste sacks for the disposal of hazardous 'soft' infectious clinical waste such as personal protective equipment (PPE), swabs and suction tips. Suspend waste sacks in a foot- or sensor-operated pedal bin. Each clinical area should have ready access to at least one pedal bin with an orange waste sack (see Figure 10.2).
- Discard waste sacks when three-quarters full, and securely tie, label and date with name of practice and premises code prior to disposal. Figure 10.5 shows the swan neck method of securing the waste bag.
- Keep manual handling of waste sacks and sharps receptacles to a minimum. Ensure that waste containers are kept upright during use or when full.
- Do not transfer waste items between clinical waste sacks.
- Return hazardous waste generated during domiciliary visits back to the practice in a yellow-lidded sharps bin or orange waste sack as appropriate, for disposal with the practice's waste.

Good practice guide: handling of hazardous waste receptacles

- Use receptacles (bins) with appropriately colour-coded lids that are rigid, puncture proof and conform to UN3291 (British Standard 7320:1990).
- Label with the premises code, description of the waste and EWC. Most sharps bins are supplied with a preprinted label containing the appropriate EWC code.
- Sharps bins should be in easy reach of the clinician, preferably wall mounted or placed on a sturdy base to prevent toppling over. The lid aperture should be in the closed position when not in use (Figure 10.6).
- Seal and dispose of containers when three-fourths full.

(a)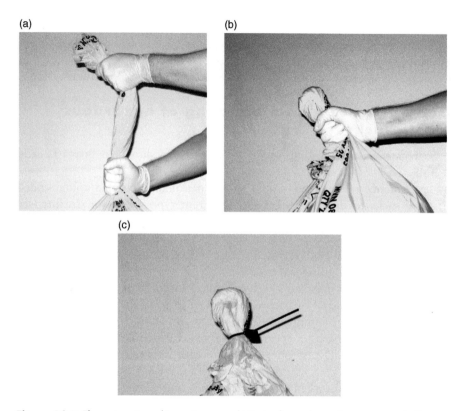

(b)

(c)

Figure 10.5 Three steps in making a 'swan neck' tie to close a hazardous waste sack. Source: Photograph kindly supplied by Dr Geoff Scott.

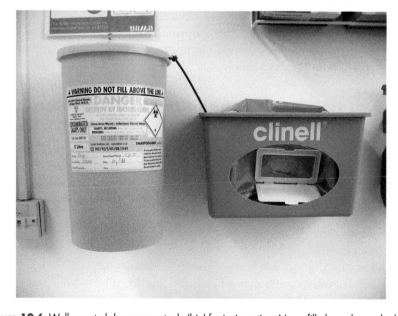

Figure 10.6 Wall-mounted sharps receptacle (bin) for incineration. Never fill above the marked line.

- Never be tempted to discharge syringes containing residual local anaesthetic solution into the sink.
- Keep sharps bins away from direct sources of heat.
- If a sharps container (or waste sack) is damaged, place inside a larger container, lock and label prior to disposal.

SAFE HANDLING OF CLINICAL WASTE PRIOR TO DISPOSAL

If those handling waste are suitably trained in the segregation and disposal of waste then according to the WHO, the actual risk of infection from healthcare waste should be minimal, except of course for sharps injuries. As a precautionary measure, any person who handles waste in the dental practice must be immunized against hepatitis B (including cleaning staff). During disposal of clinical waste, healthcare personnel should don the appropriate personal protective equipment (e.g. heavy-duty gloves and plastic apron) to protect themselves and their clothes against spills and sharps injuries. Hands should be cleaned after handling waste. If there is a risk from exposure to aerosols and splatter then masks and protective eyewear should be worn (see Chapter 6).

In the event of a sharps injury or splashing, follow the guidance described in Chapter 4, Figure 4.5. Always record the incident on an accident report form. The infection control lead is required in this situation to undertake a risk assessment, and if possible identify what went wrong, and whether a change in protocol or training could prevent similar occurrences from happening again. Such incidents often follow breaches in the local waste policy; some examples are described below.

- Sharps extruding from overfilled waste bins
- Lid of sharps bin left in open rather than closed position when not in use
- Incorrectly assembled bin
- Sharps inadvertently placed in waste sacks
- Lack of staff training
- Build-up of stored waste in an inappropriate site
- Members of the public accessing or children playing with clinical waste bins or carts
- Pest control issues

BULK STORAGE OF WASTE FOR COLLECTION

Waste carts are often heavily contaminated with pathogenic bacteria so care should always be taken to prevent escape or leakage from waste sacks or containers. It is good practice to keep a body fluid spillage kit in a convenient place close to where waste for collection is stored (see Chapter 8); if incidents do occur, they can be dealt with promptly.

Good practice guide: bulk storage of waste

- Waste should be stored in a dedicated area prior to collection.
- Clinical waste sacks and bins awaiting collection should be stored in a UN-type rigid fire-retardant locked waste cart with a well-fitting lid.
- Waste storage areas should be clean, secure, well lit and inaccessible to unauthorized persons or pests such as foxes and squirrels.
- Waste should be stored on an impervious hard surface that can be washed down should there be a spillage.
- Waste should be collected at frequent intervals to prevent a build-up of waste sacks. The actual frequency will be dictated by the volume of waste generated.
- Waste can only be stored at the dental premises for a maximum of 12 months.

TRANSPORT OF HAZARDOUS WASTE

Completing consignment notes for hazardous waste and keeping records

Every movement of hazardous waste (technically referred to as consigning) must be accompanied by a completed multipart consignment note. This must be signed at each stage during the transfer of waste from the practice to the waste disposal site. This ensures 'cradle to grave' tracking of the movement of waste and that the information accompanying the waste is sufficient to enable its safe disposal. The legal responsibility for describing the waste rests with the dental practice. A new consignment note must be completed for each individual collection of hazardous waste. Each consignment note consists of producer, carrier and consignee (waste disposal contractor) copies.

There are two different types of documentation required for waste transfers.

1. *Consignment notes*, which are used for hazardous wastes (special wastes in Scotland)
2. *Waste transfer notes*, which are used for non-hazardous wastes

Box 10.4 explains the stages involved in completing a consignment note for hazardous waste.

BENEFITS OF WASTE SEGREGATION

The stated aim of the national waste strategy is to reduce the amount of healthcare waste produced each year. Not surprisingly, the regulations are drafted in such a way as to actively encourage practices to evaluate their activities and

> ## Box 10.4 Completing consignment notes for hazardous waste
>
> - The dentist/nominated member of staff must complete their portion of the consignment note before collection and removal of the waste. Both the waste carrier and the dentist must sign the note.
> - When the premises are registered, a hazardous waste producer registration number (called a 'premises code') must be used on all consignment notes. Registration is only valid for 12 months and therefore must be renewed annually.
> - Consignment note includes the following information to prevent subsequent mismanagement of the waste:
>   - a written description of the waste
>   - EWC code
>   - quantity of waste to be consigned in kg
>   - chemical and biological components of the waste, concentration, hazard codes and the physical form of the waste, e.g. solid or liquid
>   - number, type of waste containers and their capacity
>   - any special handling requirements.
> - The waste carrier must then give a copy to both the waste producer (dental practice) and the waste disposal contractor (consignee).
> - The waste disposal contractor must send quarterly returns (evidence that the waste has been treated and disposed of correctly) to the dental practice, usually in the form of a copy consignment note. The waste contractor will also have a duty to notify the Environment Agency of the amount of hazardous waste collected, treated or disposed.
> - Practices are required to keep records of the hazardous waste they produce. Transfer notes are to be kept for two years, including those issued from a pharmacy. Consignment notes plus the return from the consignee certifying receipt of the waste are kept for a period of three years from the date the waste was removed.

explore methods to limit waste generation and curb pollution. Cost and energy savings can be made by both correct segregation of clinical waste which avoids unnecessary incineration of waste and recycling of non-clinical waste. Incineration not only contributes to global warming but also is up to 10 times more expensive than low-temperature processing. Financial penalties or even prosecutions can be imposed on those dental practices that fail to dispose of waste in the correct manner, as they are in breach of their 'duty of care'.

REFERENCES AND WEBSITES

Department of the Environment Northern Ireland. (2014) Waste Management: The Duty of Care. Approved Code of Practice for Northern Ireland. Available at: www. doeni.gov.uk/sites/default/files/publications/doe/waste-policy-duty-of-care-code-of-practice-2014.pdf (accessed 4 November 2016).

HEALTHCARE WASTE MANAGEMENT

Department of Health. (2013) HTM 07-01 Management and Disposal of Healthcare Waste. Available at: www.gov.uk/government/publications/guidance-on-the-safe-management-of-healthcare-waste (accessed 4 November 2016).

Finley RL, Collignon P, Joakim Larsson DG *et al.* (2013) The scourge of antibiotic resistance: the important role of the environment. *Clinical Infectious Diseases*, **57**, 704–710.

Human Tissue Authority (2014) Human Tissue Act. Code of Practice 1 – Consent. Available at: www.hta.gov.uk/guidance-professionals/codes-practice/code-practice-1-consent (accessed 4 November 2016).

Scottish Environment Protection Agency. Clinical Waste. Available at: www.sepa.org.uk/regulations/waste/special-waste/clinical-waste/(accessed 4 November 2016).

Chapter 11

Transport and postage of diagnostic specimens, impressions and equipment for servicing and repair

The transport of infectious items sent by post or courier (e.g. diagnostic clinical specimens, impressions or dental equipment requiring servicing and repair) is governed by the national and international regulations on the Carriage of Dangerous Goods by Road (ADR). These regulations are intended to prevent accidental exposure of people, vehicles or machinery to hazardous materials while a package is in transit. In this era of heightened awareness of bioterrorism, correct and safe packaging of infectious items has taken on renewed importance. Compliance with the regulations by the healthcare community is essential if airlines and courier services are to continue transporting clinical material.

National and international ADR regulations are based on the United Nations (UN) publication entitled 'Guidance on Regulations for the Transport of Infectious Substances', which are revised every two years (http://apps.who.int/iris/bitstream/10665/149288/1/WHO_HSE_GCR_2015.2_eng.pdf?ua=1). The UN classifies pathogens for the purposes of international transport into two categories, A and B (Table 11.1). Some substances, however, are not subject to this classification and the exemptions that are relevant to dentistry are outlined in this chapter.

Basic Guide to Infection Prevention and Control in Dentistry, Second Edition.
Caroline L. Pankhurst.
© 2017 John Wiley & Sons Ltd. Published 2017 by John Wiley & Sons Ltd.
Companion website: www.wiley.com/go/pankhurst/infection-prevention

Table 11.1 UN categories for the transport of infectious substances

Category	Definition	UN number	Proper shipping name
A	'An infectious substance which is transported in a form that, when exposure to it occurs, is capable of causing permanent disability, life-threatening or fatal disease in otherwise healthy humans or animals' (*based on professional judgement, known medical history and symptoms of the patient or endemic local conditions*)	UN 2814	INFECTIOUS SUBSTANCE AFFECTING HUMANS
B	'An infectious substance which does not meet the criteria for inclusion in Category A'	UN 3373	BIOLOGICAL SUBSTANCE, CATEGORY B

Source: Modified from World Health Organization. Guidance on Regulations for the Transport of Infectious Substances 2015–2016. http://apps.who.int/iris/bitstream/10665/149288/1/WHO_HSE_GCR_2015.2_eng.pdf?ua=1

COLLECTING SPECIMENS

The regulations define clinical specimens as any substance, tissue or liquid, removed from the patient for the purpose of analysis. Specimens must be placed in a leak-proof container immediately after collection, either dry or in transport medium, and the lid securely fastened. The date, patient's identifying details, type and site from which the specimen is taken must be entered on both the outside of the container and the request form. Complete the request form and supply all relevant clinical information to aid the pathologist to make a diagnosis. Then the container is placed in a plastic specimen transport bag and the accompanying request form is inserted into a *separate* pouch to avoid contamination should the specimen leak in transit.

Good practice guide: reducing the risk of cross-infection or injury when handling specimens

- Only staff trained to do so should handle specimens.
- The specimen container should be placed in the bag separately from the request form and then placed in the designated carrying box. Staples, pins or paper clips should not be used to seal or attach forms to the bag (Figure 11.1).
- Leaking and broken specimen containers should be disposed of as hazardous waste and any spillage cleaned up promptly.
- Masks, protective eyewear and gloves should be worn when taking specimens.

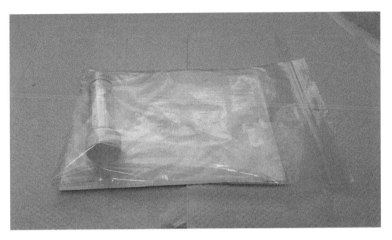

Figure 11.1 A specimen bottle (primary packaging) in a zip-lock self-sealing specimen bag (secondary packaging); note the separate outer pouch for placement of the request form.

- Hands should be thoroughly cleaned after handling specimens.
- Specimens should not be placed in areas where food is eaten or stored (e.g. kitchen fridge).

TRANSPORT OF SPECIMENS TO THE LABORATORY

Sending non-fixed diagnostic specimens

ADR classifications

According to the ADR classifications, clinical specimens taken from dental patients for diagnostic purposes are assigned to UN 3373 category B infectious substances (diagnostic or clinical specimens). Clinical samples from dental practices transferred to hospital or private laboratories should be packed according to ADR Packing Instructions P650 for road transport or the IATA packing instruction 650 for air transport. These packaging instructions are based on the use of the UN triple-package system (Figure 11.2) which is commercially available from office suppliers. Home-made packaging is to be avoided as this is unlikely to be compliant. Packaging for category B infectious substances must be capable of passing a 1.2 m drop test. This means that following a drop from a height of 1.2 m, there is no leakage from the primary receptacle and this should remain protected by the absorbent material within the secondary packaging.

The World Health Organization (WHO) recommends a basic triple-packaging system which is suitable for all infectious substances. It consists of three layers as shown in Figure 11.2.

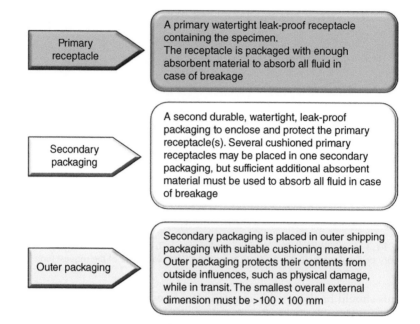

Figure 11.2 WHO triple packaging requirements.

Labelling

Outer packaging is labelled with the proper shipping name in letters at least 6 mm high, i.e. 'BIOLOGICAL SUBSTANCE CATEGORY B', and must display the symbol shown in Figure 11.2. Packages containing liquids must show package orientation labels. Copies of the paperwork should also be enclosed within the packaging plus an emergency response procedure in case of accidents. For airfreight, complete an airway bill form that is supplied by the airline. Packages should be clearly labelled with the delivery address and sender's details with emergency contact details, including a named person, at both where the package is being sent from and where it is going to, and a telephone number in case of leaks or queries.

Packages containing liquids must show package orientation labels. Failure to comply with the postal and transport packaging regulations may lead to prosecution.

TRANSPORT RESTRICTIONS

Public transport

A member of the dental team transporting clinical samples as part of their work, such as on domiciliary visits or when working at two clinics/surgeries, is expected to comply with the ADR regulations. Category B infectious substances must not be carried by a member of staff on their person or in a bag on public transport.

Similarly, infectious substances in category A or category B are not permitted for transport in carry-on or checked baggage on airlines, nor may they be carried on the person. A member of staff transporting clinical samples as part of their work would be expected to comply with the ADR regulations, whereas a dental patient is permitted to take their clinical sample to a dental surgery on public transport, as this is outside the remit of the ADR regulations.

Mail and courier services

Mail services will accept category B diagnostic specimens provided they are packaged to P650 requirements. For transport by road (private car or courier service), there are no limits on the quantity of materials allowed within either the primary receptacle(s) or the total package. This is in contrast to air transport either by passenger or by cargo aircraft where other than for body parts (or whole bodies), there is a 4 L/4 kg limit per package, with a 1 L limit per primary receptacle for liquids, whereas for solids, the primary receptacle must not exceed the outer packaging mass limit of 4 kg (International Air Transport Association: www.iata.org).

FIXED PATHOLOGICAL SPECIMENS

Several types of clinical diagnostic specimens are exempted from the ADR regulations.

- Blood specimens for biochemical tests, e.g. blood glucose levels, where it is assumed that such specimens would be free of pathogens unless the patient is a carrier of a blood-borne virus infection.
- Fixed histopathology specimens: pathogens that might have been present in the specimen are destroyed by the fixation process.

Both types of specimens are not considered to be a health risk unless they meet the criteria for inclusion in another class, for example, they contain toxic or radioactive chemicals. A condition of eligibility for the exemption criteria requires that the specimens are appropriately packaged for posting and shipping.

Packaging

Oral pathological specimens for histopathology are placed in a leak-proof container filled with formalin with a screw-top cap and then placed in a self-sealing plastic bag. Clearly label the outside of the container with the patient's name, number, date of birth and site of specimen. Most laboratories will supply you with a histopathology request form which both identifies the specimen and asks for additional clinical information to aid diagnosis. The form must be placed in a separate plastic bag or pouch from the specimen. Should the formalin leak out of the container then the patient information remains legible and the specimen can be reliably identified. The laboratory may refuse to accept a specimen they cannot identify by the request form.

The packaging must comply with the following ADR requirements to prevent any leakage occurring. The packaging consists of three components.

1. A leak-proof primary receptacle(s), e.g. screw-top bottle (Figure 11.1)
2. A leak-proof secondary packaging, e.g. leak-proof, sealed plastic bag
3. Outer packaging of adequate strength for its capacity, mass and intended use, and with at least one surface having minimum dimensions of 100×100 mm

When sending several specimens in the same packaging, individually wrap tubes/bottles or use a box with dividers to avoid breakages occurring in transit. For liquid specimens, place sufficient absorbent material between the primary receptacle(s) and the secondary packaging both to cushion the specimen from breakage and to absorb the entire volume of liquid in case of a leak. This will prevent compromising the integrity of the outer packaging and avoid contaminating persons handling the package or sorting office machinery. The outer padded leak-proof postal packet should be clearly marked with the words 'PATHOLOGICAL SPECIMEN – FRAGILE WITH CARE' and the name and address of the sender (and person to be contacted in case of leakage or queries) and that of the recipient.

TRANSPORTING IMPRESSIONS

In response to the commercial advantages of the 'global marketplace', it is not uncommon for dentists to send dental impression to laboratories overseas. Regardless of whether the impressions are sent to a laboratory in the UK or overseas, the transport and postal regulations will apply. However, if the impression is thoroughly disinfected as described in Chapter 7, then it will no longer pose an infection hazard, making it exempt under the ADR regulations for category B substances. The packaging requirements described for fixed diagnostic specimens will still apply. Packaging can be reused unless it becomes soiled or damaged.

EQUIPMENT TO BE SENT FOR SERVICE OR REPAIR

Dental equipment, which has been contaminated with blood/body fluids or has been exposed to patients with a known infectious disease, should be decontaminated before being dispatched to third parties for service or repair. The same principles apply as for diagnostic specimens, namely that the device or equipment should not expose the recipient to biological, chemical or radiation hazards. Therefore, if medical equipment is decontaminated and drained of any liquid, it is exempt from the dangerous goods regulations.

In some circumstances, it may be necessary to seek additional advice from the manufacturer on the most appropriate mode of decontamination, especially for electronic or electrical equipment. Accompanying the equipment should be a written declaration providing the following information on the contamination status of the equipment.

- It is contaminated with blood, body fluids, pathogens or hazardous chemicals – Yes/No.
- It has been cleaned and/or decontaminated – Yes/No.
- State the method used for cleaning, disinfection or sterilization.
- Signed and dated to declare that '*the item has been prepared to ensure safe handling and transportation*'.

If it is not possible to decontaminate the equipment (e.g. if it requires dismantling by an engineer in order to be able to clean the interior), then the repair company should be contacted and asked if they will accept a contaminated item. When dispatching devices via mail or courier, the shipping and packaging requirements described above will apply. If the repair company does not agree to the dispatch of the device, then quarantine the item, label with its contamination status and arrange a site visit to the practice by the company.

REFERENCES AND WEBSTES

Department of Health (2007) *Transport of Infectious Substances – Best Practice Guidance for Microbiology Laboratories*. London: Inspector of Microbiology and Infection Control, Department of Health. Available at: http://webarchive.nationalarchives.gov.uk/20130107105354/http:/www.dh.gov.uk/en/Publicationsandstatistics/Publications/PublicationsPolicyAndGuidance/DH_075439 (accessed 4 November 2016).

World Health Organization. Guidance on Regulations for the Transport of Infectious Substances 2015–2016. Available at: http://apps.who.int/iris/bitstream/10665/149288/1/WHO_HSE_GCR_2015.2_eng.pdf?ua=1 (accessed 4 November 2016).

Appendix

Table A.1 Daily infection control clinical pathway.

At the start of the day

- Remove watch and rings (except plain wedding bands). Work bare below the elbows; wash hands with soap and water
- Clean rubber door seal and chamber of sterilizer with clean, damp, non-linting cloth
- Fill the sterilizer reservoir with fresh reverse osmosis (RO) or distilled water (new bottle of commercially produced water or <12 hours old water generated on site)
- Confirm the sterilizer is working correctly by completing an automatic control test (for all types of sterilizers) and in addition a steam penetration test (for vacuum sterilizers – chamber must be empty except for test kit)
- Record and retain results of ACT (temperature, pressure and holding time and steam penetration test in sterilizer logbook; record if sterilizer passed or failed test, cycle number, sign and date)
- Check sufficient sterile instruments are available for the session. Run sterilizer as required; record cycle number in patient's notes (optional best practice)
- Don heavy-duty gloves, apron and goggles for cleaning surfaces with disinfectant and if preparing fresh solutions of detergents and disinfectants
- Disinfect with biocide the DUWL and reservoir bottle. Fill DUWL reservoir with fresh RO or distilled water. Flush lines for two minutes. Replenish biocide in waterlines if using continuous dosing biocide system
- Prepare fresh solution of detergent for ultrasonic bath, fill with solution and run bath empty for two minutes to degas bath. Clean down and replace solution in the bath at the end of the session or more often if visibly dirty
- Check all clinical surfaces are clean and free of clutter. Clean all surfaces with a hard surface disinfectant wipe. Clean chair and headrest
- Switch on air conditioning or open windows to ensure good ventilation in the dental surgery

Basic Guide to Infection Prevention and Control in Dentistry, Second Edition.
Caroline L. Pankhurst.
© 2017 John Wiley & Sons Ltd. Published 2017 by John Wiley & Sons Ltd.
Companion website: www.wiley.com/go/pankhurst/infection-prevention

Table A.1 (Continued)

In preparation for patient treatment

- Cover chair, light switches, handles, suction and air and waterlines with disposable single-use coverings. Items can be passed into 'dirty zones' but contaminated items should not be passed out into 'clean zones'
- Place sterile instrument set on the bracket table, check integrity and expiry date on packaging. To retain sterility, only open pack immediately before use on patient. Lay out other materials to be used in the 'clean zone' for the first patient. Storage containers of dental materials should not be placed in the 'dirty zone'

During patient treatment

- Recheck patient's medical history. Patient's notes, radiographs and computers should remain in the 'clean zone' and not be touched with contaminated gloved hands
- Observe standard precautions; treat all patients as potentially infectious
- Place goggles and bib on the patient
- Clean hands with alcohol-based hand rub before donning gloves and after removing gloves at the end of the procedure
- Don personal protective equipment (PPE) (apron, masks and protective eyewear then gloves). Change between patients and dispose of as infectious hazardous waste (orange waste sack)
- Reduce aerosols contamination by the use of high-volume suction and rubber dam (if appropriate)
- Work sharp safe: using safety engineered syringes and scalpels
- Clinician should dispose of single-use sharps (needles, sutures, scalpels, steel burs) into yellow-lidded sharps bin immediately after use. Only fill sharps bin to the three-quarters full level. Keep aperture of sharps bin in the closed position when not in use
- Local anaesthetic cartridges, both partially or fully discharged, are disposed of into the yellow-lidded sharps bin labeled mixed waste – sharps (18 01 03) and non-hazardous medicines (18 01 09) for incineration
- Dispose of amalgam waste in a special white-lidded mercury waste receptacle
- Remove disposable coverings at the end of treatment and dispose of as infectious hazardous waste in an orange waste sack

After treatment (wear appropriate PPE for cleaning the surgery, remove PPE before leaving treatment or decontamination area; always clean hands before and after removing gloves)

- **In treatment room**: clean and disinfect all contaminated work surfaces in the 'dirty zone'
- Rinse and disinfect impressions and other dental appliances before sending to laboratory
- Prepare surgery for next patient; flush waterlines for 20–30 seconds between patients

(Continued)

APPENDIX

Table A.1 (Continued)

- **Instrument decontamination**: transport instruments to decontamination room/area in a dedicated, clean, impermeable, rigid container with secure lid. Deposit in set-down area in 'dirty zone'
- Strictly segregate dirty from clean instruments
- Clean hands and don fresh PPE, e.g. apron, heavy-duty gloves (mask and protective eyewear if manually cleaning instruments)
- Presoak instruments in enzyme solution, foam or gel or keep instruments in a humidified environment if cannot be cleaned immediately
- Whenever possible, keep instruments together in their trays for stock control purposes (and optional instrument tracking)
- Disinfect and lubricate handpieces (preferably using an automated handpiece cleaner)
- If **manually cleaning instruments**, submerge instruments in CE-marked disinfectant made to concentration specified by manufacturer, using water at <45 °C. Scrub with a plastic long-handled brush, keeping instruments submerged, then rinse and dry using non-linting cloth and inspect with illuminated magnifier for cleanliness, function and absence of corrosion or rust
- **Ultrasonic bath** (optional): clean complex, serrated or hinged instruments in ultrasonic bath (metal instruments only, no dental handpieces). At end of cycle, rinse, dry using non-linting cloth and inspect using an illuminated magnifier
- Function testing of ultrasonic bath: to demonstrate removal of soil, once per week swab a set of instruments and test for presence of protein using a ninhydrin protein detection kit. To check if cavitation is working evenly across the bath, perform a foil ablation test or equivalent every three months. Record all test results in logbook and keep for a minimum of two years
- **Thermal washer disinfector** (TWD): preferred alternative to manual cleaning; use a thermal washer disinfector fitted with connectors for handpieces. At end of drying cycle, inspect to ensure visibly clean using magnifier. Oil handpieces as recommended by the manufacturer. Wrap instruments if using a vacuum sterilizer. Requires daily housekeeping of TWD according to manufacturer's instructions
- Once-weekly evaluation of TWD cleaning efficacy: swab and test an instrument set with ninhydrin protein detection test kit and record findings in the logbook
- Sterilize instruments at 134 °C for three minutes in vacuum or non-vacuum sterilizer; retain cycle record as a printout in the logbook or as a digital record
- **Non-vacuum sterilizer**: aseptically dry instruments, place in trays and wrap or pouch individual instruments. Dry, unwrapped instruments can be kept for one day in the surgery and used on the same day; store in clean, dry cupboard/drawer in 'clean zone' of dental surgery, reprocess if not used by the end of the day. Unwrapped instruments can be stored for up to one week in a dedicated clean storage area
- Label packs with expiry date and type of contents if not visible. Wrapped instruments can be stored for one year in clean dry environment; use first-in, first-out stock control
- Remove PPE and clean hands with alcohol hand rub or soap and water when moving from 'dirty' to 'clean zone' and on exiting the room

Table A.1 (Continued)

At the end of each session (clean hands before and after removing gloves)

- Clean and disinfect all work surfaces thoroughly in both 'dirty' and 'clean zones'
- Wipe down the dental chair, bracket table, tubing and spittoon
- Do not eat or store food or drink in the treatment or decontamination room

At the end of the day (clean hands before and after removing gloves)

- Dispose of three-quarters filled clinical waste sacks and sharps bins from treatment room and store in secure area
- Disinfect the aspirator, its tubing and the spittoon, and clean trap
- Drain down dental unit waterline and disinfect with biocide (if using an automated continuous dosing system, consult manufacturer's advice). Empty and disinfect reservoir bottle; store dry and inverted
- Drain down and clean ultrasonic bath, and leave dry
- Clean sterilizer chamber with damp, non-linting cloth, dry, leave empty with door open
- Empty and drain sterilizer water reservoir; clean and leave dry
- Dispose of any partially used bottles of water as they will be contaminated
- Change out of tunic/uniform and launder daily

Note: This is a basic outline only; please read relevant book chapter and consult national guidelines for more detailed protocols.

Table A.2 Decontamination methods for specific instruments and items of dental equipment.

Item	Decontamination requirements
Airways and endotracheal tubes	Single-use items. Any reusable items should be steam sterilized
Bracket table and handle	Cover with cling film during use; then disinfect with surface disinfectant wipe
Brushes (for cleaning equipment)	Either single use and discard or if reusable, clean with detergent. Store dry with the head upwards. Replace regularly
Burs (diamond, tungsten carbide)	Immerse in enzymic disinfectant; follow manufacturer's instructions on dilution and immersion time. Steam sterilize
Burs (steel)	Steel burs are a single-use item
Carpets	Not suitable for clinical areas. In non-clinical areas vacuum daily. Steam clean periodically
Curing light and tip	Cover tip with cling film or impervious plastic sleeve. (Tips are also available as sterilizable or as single-use disposable.) Wipe outer casing with surface disinfectant wipe after use on each patient
Dappens pot	Glass pot: clean and steam sterilize Plastic pot: single-use disposable

(Continued)

Table A.2 (Continued)

Item	Decontamination requirements
Dental chair and stools	Covering should be intact. Cover headrest with impermeable barrier (plastic wrap) and change between patients. Wipe down with disinfectant surface wipe (or as recommended by chair manufacturer) after every patient. Blood/body fluid splashes should be cleaned immediately with chlorine-releasing surface wipe (0.1%/1000 ppm). Note: Soft furnishings may be damaged by chlorine-releasing agents so check with the manufacturer for their recommended disinfectant
Dental chair switches	Cover with cling film; change between patients and disinfect with surface disinfectant wipe
Dental handpieces and connectors	Dental handpiece: automatic cleaning method is preferred to manual cleaning, e.g. automated handpiece cleaner/lubricator or thermal washer disinfector (if tolerant). Pre-oil according to handpiece manufacturer's instructions prior to placement in vacuum (or non-vacuum) sterilizer Connectors: cover handpiece couplings with single-use impervious sleeve/cling film during treatment; at end of patient treatment, remove sleeve, clean connector with surface disinfectant, replace with new sleeve
Endodontic instruments	Files and reamers are single use only. If manufactured as reusable, can be disinfected, sterilized, stored separately and reused on the same patient during the course of a multivisit RCT; discarded as hazardous sharps waste at the end of the course of treatment
Extracted teeth to be used for educational purposes	Remove amalgam restorations from the teeth and dispose into amalgam hazardous waste receptacle, label as 18 01 10. Preferably autoclave or disinfect teeth in a fresh solution of impression disinfectant, rinse in sterile or purified water (sterile water is recommended to prevent recontamination and bacterial growth and spoilage during storage), dry. Store in a leak-proof container
Face bows	Remove debris and clean with surface disinfectant; steam sterilize the fork
Fan (mechanical) and air conditioning	Avoid use of fans in clinical areas as difficult to clean effectively. If use is considered essential, then routinely wipe clean with detergent. Regularly change filters and clean air conditioning units
Furniture and fittings	Should be in good repair and all coverings intact. Choose furniture upholstered with wipeable fabrics. Damp-dust regularly with warm water and detergent. If known contamination with blood-borne virus, disinfect with chlorine-releasing wipe. Note: Soft furnishings may be damaged by chlorine-releasing agents

Table A.2 (Continued)

Item	Decontamination requirements
Forceps	Manual cleaning and ultrasonic bath or thermal washer disinfector; steam sterilize; store in clean, dry container/tray. Preferably sterilized in pouches in a vacuum sterilizer
Kidney dishes	Manual cleaning or use of thermal washer disinfector, steam sterilize; or use single-use disposables
Keyboard (computer)	Cover with cling film (plastic wrap) and change between patients or cover with a custom-made reusable vinyl/plastic keyboard cover and clean and disinfect using a disinfectant wipe between patients. Alternatively, use a washable keyboard
Light handles	Cover with cling film/impermeable cover and replace between patients. Clean with surface disinfectant after each patient
Masks	Single-use disposable
Matrix bands	Single-use disposable
Metal syringes	Automated cleaning in a thermal washer disinfector or manually cleaning followed by steam sterilization. Plastic syringes are single use only
Mouse (computer)	Do not touch with contaminated gloved hands. Use headrest cover as an overglove or use a washable mouse
Nail brushes	Single use only (generally not recommended for hand hygiene in dental practice)
Needles	Single-use item. Use safety engineered needles. Dispose of plastic syringes and needles as one unit into yellow-lidded sharps bin
Plastic aprons	Single use
Paper points	Use presterilized packs
Radiographic film	Handle with gloves; use barrier pouch
Radiographic film holders and positioning devices	Sterilize; if not heat tolerant then clean by immersion in disinfectant
Radiograph tube – heads and control panels	Protect with cling film (impervious barrier); change after each patient
Soft toys	Not suitable for dental surgeries as they cannot be disinfected effectively
Spittoon	Clean outer surface first. Inner surface of bowl – add (metered) dose of non-foaming disinfectant, wipe evenly around inside of bowl, leave for time interval specified by manufacturer, rinse with bowl flush and then discard disinfection cloth
Stethoscopes	Use disinfectant wipes on bell and earpieces
Suction tips	Disposable suction tips, single use only

APPENDIX

(Continued)

Table A.2 (Continued)

Item	Decontamination requirements
Suction lines	Trap filters must be removed and cleaned every night with a non-foaming disinfectant and rinsed thoroughly before replacing. Do not use bleach or hypochlorite with a metal filter as it causes rusting. Tubing and lines should be disinfected with a non-foaming disinfectant/detergent and left overnight as specified in manufacturer's instructions
Thermometer	High-level disinfection according to manufacturer's instructions or use disposable strips. DO NOT AUTOCLAVE as contains mercury
Ultrasonic scalers and handle	Scalers are steam sterilized. Cover handles in cling film or impervious plastic sleeve which is changed after each patient and wipe connector and hose with surface disinfectant

Note: The list is not exhaustive. See relevant book chapter or national guidelines for more detailed advice.

Table A.3 Examples of hand and hard surface disinfectants and dental unit waterline biocides.

Type of disinfectant/ antiseptic	Proprietary name	Use in dental surgery
Chlorhexidines		
Chlorhexidine gluconate liquid 4%	Hibiscrub surgical scrub	Hand washing
Chlorhexidine 2.5% in 70% alcohol solution in a glycerine base	Hibisol hand rub	Hand rub
Chlorhexidine 0.5% in 70% alcohol	Alcoholic chlorhexidine	Skin disinfection prior to perioral biopsy, implant surgery and periodontal surgery
Chlorhexidine gluconate 0.12% and ethanol 12%	Lines	Biocide for disinfection of dental unit waterlines and reservoir bottles
Iodophors		
	Betadine surgical scrub	Hand washing
Iodine filtration cartridge	Dentapure	Dental unit waterline biocide
Alcohols		
Alcohol gel/solutions	Purell, Sterillium, Desderman	Hand rub

Table A.3 (Continued)

Type of disinfectant/ antiseptic	Proprietary name	Use in dental surgery
70% Isopropyl alcohol wipes	Azowipes or Cliniwipes	Surgery hard surface disinfection or external surface of handpieces
Ethanol and 1-propanol alcohol spray	Mikrozoid	Surgery hard surface disinfection
Chlorine-releasing agents		
Sodium dichloroisocyanurate solution tablets 4.75 g (=2.5 g available chlorine) or granules	Haz-tabs tablet or granules Presept tablets or granules	Spillage of blood or other body fluids
Sodium hypochlorite + detergent	Chloros	Surgery hard surface disinfection
Chlorine dioxide	Tristel (chlorine dioxide-releasing wipes	Surgery hard surface disinfection
Chlorine dioxide	Microclear	Biocide for disinfection of dental unit waterlines
Triclosan		
Triclosan 2%	Aquasept	Hand disinfection
Triclosan	Skinsan	Waterless hand disinfection foam
Phenolics		
Hycolin 2% solution	Stericol, Clearsol	These products contain 2,4,6-trichlorophenol and/or xylenol, which were not supported under a recent biocides review. As such, these products can no longer be supplied for any application in the UK
Peracetic acid		
Peracetic acid	Nu-cidex Gigasept PA	High-level disinfection of heat-sensitive equipment, *only* for intermediate- and low-risk procedures

(Continued)

Table A.3 (Continued)

Type of disinfectant/ antiseptic	Proprietary name	Use in dental surgery
Superoxidized water		
Electrolysed salt solution produced by a dedicated generator (releases oxidizing agents and chlorine)	Sterilox	Biocide for disinfection of dental unit waterlines and reservoir bottles
Alkaline peroxide based		
Alkaline peroxide (plus QAC)	Sterilex Ultra	Biocide for disinfection of dental unit waterlines and reservoir bottles
Hydrogen peroxide, silver ions	Dentisept P, Oxygenal 6, Sanosil Super 25	
Citric acid based		
Sodium hypochlorite, citric acid	Alpron	Biocide for disinfection of dental unit waterlines and reservoir bottles
Quaternary ammonium compounds (QAC)		
QAC plus polymeric hexamethyl biguanide	Clinell wipes, Mikrozid alcohol-free wipes, Continu wipes	Hard surface surgery disinfectant and general-purpose wipe
QAC plus alkaline cleaning agents	Orotol plus	Suction tubing disinfectant

Note: The list contains examples only and is not exhaustive.

FURTHER SOURCES OF INFORMATION

A list of key national and international organizations that produce policy documents, advice and information relating to infection control and prevention is available on the companion website www.wiley.com/go/pankhurst/infection-prevention. They have been arranged alphabetically according to geographical region.

Index

Note: Italicized page numbers refer to figures and tables

acrylonitrile, *88t*
aerosols, 25, 81, *91t*, 162–4
alcohol based hand rubs, 71–6
alkaline peroxide, 175, *216t*
amalgam separators, 193–4
amalgam waste, *190t*, 193–4
anatomical waste, 191
anti-discrimination legislation, 51
antimicrobial
  resistance, 8
  stewardship, 8–9
approved control of practice (ACOP), 8,
    179–80
aspirators, 161
autoclaving, *189f*
automatic control test, 134–5, *208t*
avian flu, 26–7

back siphonage, 177
biocides, 175–6, *212t*
biofilms, 147, 167–8
blood-borne viruses (BBV), 22–5
  exposure-prone procedures, 47–50
  hepatitis B virus, 22–3
  hepatitis C virus, 23–4
  human immunodeficiency
      virus, 24–6
  post-exposure prophylaxis, 62–6
  preventing infection in occupational
      setting, 22
  risk factors for exposure, *63t*
  transmission of, 52–5
blood spills, cleaning, 164–6

body fluid spillages, cleaning, 164–6
B-type sterilizers, 130–2

cardiopulmonary resuscitation,
    protection during, 97
care quality commission (CQC), 8
chemical process indicators, 136–7
chlorhexidine gluconate, *175t*
chlorine releasing agents, 164, *212t*
citric acid, *175t*
cleaning, 154–6
  cleaning plan, 154–5
  national colour code155–6
clean room/zone, 112
clinical governance, 13, 66
clinical waste, 182–7, 189–93, 197
cold sterilization, 144–5
communicable diseases, 16–28
  emerging/re-emerging pathogens, 28–9
  sources of infection, 16–17
  transmission routes, 18–22
    airborne, 25
    blood stream, 22–5
    direct and indirect contact, 20
community-acquired MRSA
    (CA-MRSA), 20–2
compressors, 12
Control of Substances Hazardous to
    Health Regulations 2002, 10–11
Creutzfeldt-Jakob disease and vCJD,
    29–32, 106–7, 143–4
  sngle use instruments, 144
cross infection, 1–2, 17–19

Basic Guide to Infection Prevention and Control in Dentistry, Second Edition.
Caroline L. Pankhurst.
© 2017 John Wiley & Sons Ltd. Published 2017 by John Wiley & Sons Ltd.
Companion website: www.wiley.com/go/pankhurst/infection-prevention

decontamination, 105–10
  cycle, 105–6
  facility, 110–16
    basic requirements, *116t*
    design of, 110–15
    sterile instrument storage,
      139–40
    temporal separation, 115–16
  legal requirements, 107–8
  location, 110
  for specific instruments, *211–14t*
  technical standards, 109–10
deionised water, 132–3
delayed hypersensitivity, 89
dental chair, 149–50
dental equipment
  decontamination methods,
    211–14t
  heat-sensitive, 144–6
  purchasing of, 117–8
  for service or repair, 201, 206–7
  type A airgap, *174t*
dental handpieces, cleaning of,
    22, 145–6
dental impressions, disinfection
    of, 123–4
dental instruments, 22, 105–6
  automated versus manual
    cleaning, 118
  decontamination requirements,
    211–14t
  inspection, 130
  manual cleaning of, 119–21
  out of hours use, 141–2
  passive layer, 119
  presterilization cleaning of, 118
  preventing corrosion of, 118
  risk assessment, *109t*
  single-use, 119–20
  sterilization of, 130
  stock control, 141
  traceability of, 141
  unwrapped, storage of, 139–40
dental practice, risk assessment in, 4–6
dental surgery design, 148–53
  clinical waste, 152
  dental chair, 150
  flooring, 150
  lighting, 150–1
  protective clothing, 153
  room size, 149
  sharp containers, 152
  storage of equipment and chemicals,
    152–3
  ventilation, 153
  washbasins, 151
  work surfaces and zoning, 149
dental unit waterlines, 22, 25, 167–73
  biocides, 173–6
  biofilms, 167–8, *215–16t*
  control of legionella in, 179–80
  decontamination of, 173–81
  health risks from, 168–73
    endotoxin, 173
    legionellae, 170–1
    mycobacterium, 172
    prevention of backsiphonage, 177
    pseudomonads, 171–2
    sterile irrigation 178
Department of Environment, Food and
    Rural Affairs, 184
dermatitis, 82–4
disinfectants, *214–16t*
disinfection
  dental handpieces, 121
  dental impression, 146
  hard surfaces, 144
  heat sensitive equipment, 144
distilled water, 132–3

ebola virus, 18, 28–9, 51, 93
emerging pathoens, 28–9
emollient hand cream, 83–4
endotoxin, 106, 129, 132, 173
Environment Agency, 184, 199
Epstein-Barr virus (HBV), 21
European waste catalogue codes, *184t*,
    187t, 189–93
exposure-prone procedures (EPPs),
    47–50

face shields, 95–7
failures
  active, 36
  latent, 36–7
flooring, 156

gasification, *188f*
general cleaning, 154–5
General Dental Council (GDC)
  standards, 51
gloves, 86–91
  allergy to, 88–90
  aseptic removal, *98f*
  choosing, 88
  heavy duty, 82, *115f*, 197
  properties of, *88t*
  role of, 86–7
  safe use in dental surgery, 87
goggles, 85, 95–7

hand creams, 83–4
hand hygiene, 68–84
  products, 81–2, *214t*
  and team working, 70–5
  techniques, 76–82
    alcohol based hand rubs, 71–6, 80
    removing rings and watches76
    standard technique, 76–81
    surgical hand washing, 89
  washbasins, 81–2
hands
  care of, 82–3
  emollient hand cream, 83–4
  microbial colonisation of, 68
  prevention of irritant dermatitis, 82–3
  resident bacteria, 68–9
  as source of hospital-acquired
    infection, 69–70
  transient bacteria, 68–9
  when to clean, 70, *74f*
Hazardous Waste Regulations 2005, 183
hazardous wastes, 183, *184t*, 185–90
  alternative non-burn processes, *189f*
  amalgam waste, 193–4
  anatomical waste, 191
  bulk storage, 197–8
  clinical waste, 190–1
  consignment notes, 198–9
  dental healthcare waste streams,
    184–5
  European waste catalogue
    codes, *187t*
  extracted teeth, 191
  high temperature processes, *188f*

legislation, 182–4
low temperature processes, *189f*
prescription only medicines waste,
  192–3
radiographic, 193
safe handling and storage of, 195–7
segregation and disposal of, 197–8
transfer notes, 198
transport of, 198
types of, 189–90
Health and Safety at Work Act 1974,
  9–10, 51, 85
Health and Social Care Act approved
  code of practice, 7–8, *9t*
health care-associated infections
  (HCAIs), 18–19
health care workers (HCWs), 46
health clearance, 38, 46–51
  additional health checks/clearance,
    48–50
  duty of care, 50–1
  standard health checks, 46–7
health technical memorandum
  (HTM), 13
  HTM 01–05, 107–10
  HTM 07–01, 183–4
heat-sensitive equipment, disinfection of,
  144–6, *215t*
hepatitis viruses
  hepatitis B immunoglobulin (HBIG),
    43, *65t*
  hepatitis B vaccine, 43–5, 64–6
  hepatitis B virus, 18, 22–3
  hepatitis C virus, 18, 23–4
  herpes simplex virus (HSV), 18–21
human immunodeficiency virus (HIV),
  24–5, 50, 54–5, 60–1
hypersensitivity, 83, 89–90

immediate hypersensitivity, 83, 89
immunisation programme, 39–46
  hepatitis B, 43–5
  measles mumps and rubella (MMR),
    39–41
  tuberculosis, 42–3
  varicella, 41–2
incineration, 182, *185f*, 186–8
index case, 18

infection, 19–29
  emerging/re-emerging pathogens, 28–9
  route, 19–20
  transmission, 20–3
  control, 1–15
    daily, clinical pathway, *208–11t*
    laws, 7–12
    policy, 12
    procedures, 13
    risk assessment, 3–7
    standards and guidance, 12–13
    team approach, 13–5
influenza, 26–7
iodophors, *72t, 214t*
irritant dermatitis, 82–3

latex allergies, 88
latex-free environment, 88–9
legionellae, 170–2
Legionnaires' disease, patients at risk of,
    171t
  Legionnaires' disease: The control of
    legionella bacteria in water
    systems. Approved Code of
    Practice L8, *174t, 179t*, 180

macrowaves, *189f*
masks, 91–5
  best practice guide, 92
  as personal protective equipment, 92
  respirator, 94–5
  respiratory hygiene, 95
  surgical, 91–3
Medical Devices Regulations 2002,
    105–7
methicillin-resistant *Staphylococcus
    aureus* (MRSA), 18–19
microfibre cloths, 155
microwaving, *189f*
mouthpieces, 97–8
mouth-to-mouth resuscitation,
    protection during, 97–8
mycobacterium, *145t*, 146
  BCG, 25–6, *40t*, 45–6
  in DUWL, 169, 172

natural rubber latex, 88–90
needles, 54–60

resheathing of, *58f*
safe disposal of, 59–60
safe handling of, 56–8
safety needles, 58–9
N-type sterilizers, 130–1

occupational health, 34–52
  anti-discrimination legislation, 50
  exposure-prone procedures, 47–8
  health clearance, 46–7
  immunisation programme,
    39–45
  pre-employment health assessment,
    46–7
  risk activities in dentistry, 34
  safety culture, 35–7
  staff health records, 37–9
  women of childbearing
    age, 39–43
opportunist pathogens, 16–7

pandemic influenza, 27
peracetic acid, 145, *175t, 215t*
percutaneous transmission, 22
personal protective equipment
    (PPE), 85–6
  face shields, 95–7
  gloves, 86–8
  goggles, 95–7
  masks, 91–5
  plastic aprons, 102–4
  putting on, 97
  removing, 97
  respirator masks, 94–5
  surgical gowns, 104
phenolic, *215t*
plasma technology, *188f*
plastic aprons, 102–4
pocket resuscitation masks, 97
polychloroprene, *88t*
pre-employment health assessment, 38
prescription only medicines
    waste, *190t*, 192–3
Pressure Systems Safety Regulations
    2000, 11–12
protective clothing, 85–6
protective eyewear, 95–7, 197, 202
protein detection test, 126–8

Pseudomonas infection, 171–2
purified water, 132–3
pyrolysis, *188f*

Reporting of Injuries, Diseases and
    Dangerous Occurrences
    Regulations, 7, 11
respirator masks, 26, 91, 93–5
respiratory hygiene, 95
respiratory syncytial virus (RSV), 95
risks, 2–6
    assessment of, 4–6
    management, 6–7
    relative risks, 2
rubella, 21, 39–41

safety culture, 35–7
safety sharps, 58–9
saliva ejectors, 161–2
severe acute respiratory syndrome
    (SARS), 30, 93, 95
sharp containers, *57t*, 152
sharps injuries, 53–66
    accident risk assessment, 66
    avoiding, 56–67
    blood-borne virus infections, 53–6
    hepatitis C exposures, 62–4
    managing, 60–2
    occurrence, 55
    post-exposure prophylaxis, 64–6
    preventable, 56
    recording of, 66
    resheathing needles, 57
        safe disposal of sharps and needles,
        59–60
        safe handling of sharps and needles,
        56–60
        use of safety devices, 56–9
        risk assessment for BBV exposure,
        62–4
sharp instruments in healthcare
    regulations 2013, *57t*
single-use instruments, 142–4
    consequences of reuse, 142–4
    quality of, 143
    rationale for, 144
    and variant Creutzfeldt-Jakob
        disease, 144

specimens, 202–6
    collecting, 202–3
    fixed pathological, 205–6
    legal framework, 201
    mail and courier services, 205
    non-fixed diagnostic, 203–4
    public transport of, 204
    transport restrictions, 204–5
    transport to laboratory, 204–5
    waste disposal, 191
spittoons, 161
splatter, 162–4
standard hand hygiene technique, 76–80
standard infection control precautions
    (SICPs), 18
steam auger, *189f*
steam penetration test, 135–6
sterilization, 130–42
    of heat sensitive instruments, 144–5
    instrument traceability, 141–2
    storage of unwrapped instruments,
        139–40
sterilizers, 130–40
    installation of, 131
    loading, 130, 138
    operating, 11–12, 109, 116–17,
        208–11t
    pressure, 134
    suitability of, 130–1
    storage of instruments, 138–40
    temperature, 134
    testing, 133–6
        automatic control test, 134–5
        chemical process indicators, 136–7
        failures, 135
        periodic testing, 133–4
        steam penetration test, 135–6
    validation of, 131
    water reservoir, 132–3
        biofilm formation in, 132
        maintenance of, 133
        recycled water, 133
        steam purity, 132
        types of water, 132–3
S-type sterilizers, 131
superoxidized water, *216t*
surface cleaning, 156–60
surgical gowns, 104

surgical hand washing, *73t*, 81
syphilis, 43

thermal washer disinfectors, 107, 122,
     126–30
transmissible spongiform
     encephalopathy, 30–2
triclosan, *72t*, 75, *215t*
tuberculosis, 18, 25–6, 34, *40t*, 93
tunics, 45–6

ultrasonic baths, 124–6, *128f*
uniforms, 99–101
universal precautions, 18
unwrapped instruments, storage of, 138–40

vaccinations, *40t*
varicella, immunisation and vaccination,
     41–2

varicella zoster virus (VZV), 21
ventilation, 153
vinyl, *88t*, *213t*
visors, 95–7

wash hand basins, 151–2
water reservoir chamber, 132–3
women of childbearing age, 39–43
   risks from rubella, 41
   risks from syphilis, 43
   risks from varicella, 41–2
   varicella immunisation/
        vaccination, 39
World Health Organization,
     41, 70

Zika virus, 19–20, 28
zoning, 156–60
zoonosis, 29–32

Printed and bound by CPI Group (UK) Ltd, Croydon, CR0 4YY

09/10/2024

14571429-0003

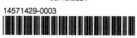